W9-BBA-777

Chronic Crisis:

Critical Care for America's

Collapsing Healthcare

System

Selvoy M. Fillerup, MD, MSPH, FACS

Second Edition
ISBN: 987-0-9792531-9-5

Published by Acacia Publishing, Inc.
Phoenix, Arizona
acaciapublishing.com

To contact Dr. Fillerup, to schedule him as a speaker to your civic, social, or political group, or to purchase additional copies of *Chronic Crisis*, visit chroniccrisis.com or contact the publisher.

Cover design by Cynthia Ergenbright
www.cynergiecreations.com

Graphics by Ryan Davis
www.rybreadstudio.com

Printed and bound in Canada

chroniccrisis.com

Imagine that you never again had to worry about having healthcare coverage — for your spouse, for your child, or for yourself. That is what this book is really about.

When you have finished reading this book, go ahead and write your Senators and Congressional Representatives. You can't afford not to.

To Ruth, Kristen and Jocelyn

Table of Contents

Prologue

"Total health expenditures are estimated to be $2.16 trillion in 2006 up from $1.7 trillion in 2005, and are projected to rise to over $4 trillion in 2015. Per person health spending is $7,110 this year and is projected to increase to $12,320 by the end of the period."[1] Our existing health care financing system is financially unsustainable.

The United States health care financing system is in desperate need of a major overhaul and in 2006 has reached a pivotal point in the history of the health insurance concept.

Historically, every thirty years or so, a major change occurs in the U.S. health care financing system. Examples of two major changes are:

- *Development of the health insurance concept dominance 1940s - 1970s, and*

- *Development of the HMO/Managed Care Concept ñ dominance 1973 - 2006*

- *The question is "What will be the next health care financing quantum shift?*

Presently, the Federal Government and the private health insurance sector in the U.S. are promoting Health

Savings Accounts (HSAs), Consumer-Driven Health Plans and High Deductible Health Plans as the next innovative financing solution. These <u>financial solutions</u> only solve <u>financial</u> <u>problems</u> and will not solve our health insurance problems; they will only serve to further exacerbate the U. S. health care financing crisis.

Selvoy M. Fillerup, MD, FACS new book, ***Chronic Crisis: Critical Care for America's Collapsing Healthcare System*** describes a health insurance solution for U. S. health insurance problems. A primer, the book is written in layperson's terms that reviews a financing reform strategy using federal government oversight and a multi-payor private health insurance market to solve our health care financing problems and simultaneously improve the quality of health care services.

Dr. Fillerup takes the reader on an international journey that identifies and explains how other countries around the world handle their health care financing challenges and problems. For example, ***Did you know that a <u>majority</u> of European countries use the private health insurance market through a multi-payor system to finance their health care services and control costs rather than a single payor system?***

Dr. Fillerup's Multi-Payor Reform Strategy provides the type of political, financial and advocacy compromises that are necessary to solve the U. S. health care financing problems on a long-term basis.

The following table envisions the U.S. health care financing system in terms of a continuum — on the left side is the traditional private health insurance system and on the right side is the single payor financing (advocacy) system. The politically acceptable middle (compromise) is occupied by the Multi-Payor Reform Strategy.

The U.S. Health Care Financing Continuum:		
Private Health Insurance System (HMOs/ PPOs/ Managed care)	Multi-payer Reform Strategy	Single Payer Government Financing System

The Single Payor Financing Model, where the government is the sole payor, is too extreme for the business community to accept. Therefore, in order to accomplish universal healthcare in a cost containing environment, we find ourselves in a political no man s land between the status quo and the extreme position of single payor advocacy. What we seek is a cost effective financing model and what can be realistically accomplished.

The business and health insurance communities want to control health care costs while retaining the highest quality health care services; alternatively the single payor advocacy financing community wants a more cost effective financing system and universal affordable health care for all Americans.

Dr. Fillerup's book ***Chronic Crisis: Critical Care for America's Collapsing Healthcare System*** is the viable political compromise and blueprint that provides:

- *The business and insurance communities with the ability to control costs while retaining high quality health care services, and*

- *Single payor Advocacy groups with a more cost effective financing system assuring Universal Affordable Health Care for All.*

After you read ***Chronic Crisis: Critical Care for America's Collapsing Healthcare System***, mail it to your Senators and Congressperson with a note asking them to read it.

Thomas J. Garvey, MHA
Chairman, Board of Directors
The Center for Health Care
Policy, Research and Analysis
15 Argyle Road
Merrick, NY 11566
(516) 379-6812
http://www.thepolicy-center.org

---

1. *C. Borger et al., "Health spending projections through 2015: changes on the horizon," Health Affairs Web Exclusive, March/April 2006; 25(2): 61-73.*

Introduction

Getting to Universal Healthcare in the United States

I did not know it at the time, but this book began when I attended a symposium on the lessons the United States could learn from the Canadian healthcare experience. At that meeting I realized the grasp that past events have on peoples' perceptions. As I listened to the long recitation about the developmental steps in the United States and Canadian healthcare systems, I thought how distantly removed these historic developments seemed from the basic theoretical concepts I had learned while studying healthcare policy.

What I was hearing was how the U.S. healthcare system had developed piece by piece, dealing with one circumstance after another, and how, on the other hand, the Canadian system had been organized in one legislative moment but had then gone through a series of iterations until its present form — which continues to have troubles. The results are the collage of dysfunctional components we currently have in the U.S.

and the single-payer healthcare system with long waiting lists in Canada today. Both systems are up and running; neither system is perfect. Both systems have troubles with access: the U.S. with a significant portion of the population having no healthcare coverage, and Canada having prolonged waiting times for procedures.

The solution for the U.S. lies not in patching up the problems in existing agencies but in developing a unified healthcare policy unique to the situation of the U.S., with foundations in basic economic principles.

I spent fifteen years of my career as a practicing ear, nose and throat surgeon in a rural setting before I changed careers and studied Public Health. I did not experience HMOs; I never experienced the management complexities associated with managed care systems. The result is that my perspective of healthcare systems wanders toward theory and "the basics" rather than toward the negotiations and politics I now see my urban colleagues experiencing on a daily basis.

Having emerged from my rural environment, and having taken up the study of Public Health and U.S. healthcare policy with fresh eyes, I feel rather like a curious traveler who comes upon an inefficient village, sees its workings, and wonders why things in this village do not improve. Surrounding villages up and down the road have life's problems sufficiently under control, and there is ample communication between the villages, but somehow the forces of tradition or personal bias keep this particular village from adopting any of the methods of its neighbors. I have recently become aware that there is a new name for this institutional inertia — this hypnotic love of the status quo; it is "path dependency."[1] On one level it makes no sense at all; at another level it has its own logic.

But a "status quo" this dysfunctional is not sustainable. Social and economic forces will eventually catch up with this much inefficiency — change is certain. My point in all this is that when those changes arrive, they ought to be based on the demonstrated successes of previous experience, on applied basic business and economic theory and not simply on emotional bias or morally motivated politics. The success of moral endeavors still depends upon the correct application of basic principles — including economic principles. "Every mission has a margin; no margin, no mission."

Pragmatism trumps everything. Surgical textbooks, when describing the treatment for any surgical disease, have a section describing past surgical methods. This recitation of previous surgical techniques serves to emphasize the realities of basic anatomy, basic physiology, basic pathology and basic surgical method. Successful new techniques invariably rely on basic science, basic physics, anatomy, and physiology. Similarly, successful businesses rely on basic accounting methods, basic marketing strategies, and basic manufacturing principles to achieve success. Even though healthcare policy makers may still be on a learning curve for what those basics really are, the attainment of a successful universal healthcare system should likewise be founded on basics: basic health principles, basic business principles, and basic economic principles. Without reliance upon the basics, it is difficult to imagine a successful universal healthcare policy.

Does the U.S. need universal healthcare? The answer is emphatically yes! An inefficient status quo is not sustainable; its foundation is built on sand. The hidden costs, both social and economic, born by U.S. citizens because they lack universal healthcare far outweigh the costs of insuring all citizens. Those hidden costs will continue to mount, and eventually the unsteady foundation of the current healthcare system will collapse.

But it is reasonable to contemplate a solid foundation and a sustainable healthcare system built upon a foundation of correct principles. The first necessity is vision. Many in this country already have a vision of universal healthcare, usually of a single-payer system. But there is always the opportunity to widen one's vision and include alternatives to single-payer healthcare systems. The second necessity is policy. What policy? Citizens have a right to expect of their government a defined national healthcare policy. Health is no longer a given; new diseases present themselves at a rate of ten per year. Access to healthcare is not automatic; fifteen percent of the U.S. population is without health insurance. Many will not change employment; they persist, frozen in unproductive jobs for fear of losing healthcare benefits — in "job lock."

The third necessity is a plan. There is no one right plan, but several countries do have workable plans. And the United States certainly has the capacity to develop a plan unique to itself using the successes and failures of other plans as guides.

Once citizens recognize the secondary social benefits of universal healthcare, they will almost surely demand a comprehensive universal healthcare policy. There will be a universal healthcare system in the future of the United States. It is simply a matter of time.

You can contact Congress to convey your opinions and make your preferences known at www.congress.org.

Selvoy M. Fillerup, MD, MSPH, FACS

CHAPTER ONE

Bleeding Out

The United States' healthcare system has failed — and Americans are paying the price in terms of both dollars and ill health.

The number and percentage of the United States population without healthcare access continue to rise. Simply because they lack access to healthcare, an estimated 18,000 people die prematurely each year.[2]

Technical advances fail to reach many who need them, mostly because 15.7% of the population has no health insurance.[3]

Per capita healthcare costs in the United States, including the costs for those without health insurance, are higher than in any other industrialized nation and are 2.4 times higher than the average per capita cost for other nations in the Organization for Economic Cooperation and Development (OECD) and continue to rise.[4,5] Yet among all nations, the United States ranks 17th in life expectancy and 31st in infant mortality rates.[6]

Data published by the U.S. Centers for Disease Control and Prevention revealed the total number of uninsured Americans increased by 6 percent from 2005 to 2006. The number of uninsured adults jumped by 2 million persons during the same period.[3]

The ability of many people to obtain healthcare coverage is hampered by their employment status, by the willingness of their employer to provide health benefits, by cost, or by their current health status. Roughly half of insured Americans get their health insurance through an employment-sponsored plan, but participation in these plans is not mandatory and businesses are not legally required to offer health insurance. Thirty-seven percent of businesses with fewer than 200 employees did not offer health benefits to their employees in 2004. Even when businesses do offer health benefits, some recent employees and part time employees are not considered eligible for these plans, and some employees do not enroll because the premiums are too costly.[7]

Private non-group insurance premiums are based on individual health risk and are substantially more expensive than group plans purchased by employers, with cost varying by age and health status. Insurance companies in the non-group market can deny or limit coverage to persons in poor health or with chronic conditions.[7]

When people do not have health insurance they are more likely to forego primary healthcare or even fail to fill a needed prescription. They are less likely to receive preventive care and are more likely to become hospitalized for avoidable health problems. Insured non-elderly adults are at least 50% more likely to have had preventive care such as pap smears, mammograms, and prostate exams compared to uninsured adults. Simply having health insurance has been shown to improve overall health and could reduce mortality rates among the uninsured by 10 to 15%.[7]

In other words, many people who need health insurance in the United States cannot get it, and thousands of Americans are becoming ill or dying as a result. Yet the profits of insurance companies and HMOs continue to rise.

According to Weiss Ratings reported in *South Florida Business Journal*, August 8, 2005:

> *"Profits for the nation's health maintenance organizations increased a healthy 10.7 percent last year, with earnings reaching a total of $11.4 billion, up from $10.3 billion the year before. An insurer based in South Florida is among the leading gainers."* One particular health plan reported its net income grew from $61.6 million in 2003 to $164.9 million last year, a 168 percent change. [8]

With the healthcare market in such disarray, Americans would do well to ask some hard questions, return to basic principles of how markets function, and look beyond their own borders for pragmatic answers.

Lessons From Abroad

In the United States, per capita healthcare costs are higher than in any other nation.[5] The obvious question is "why?" What, exactly, makes the United States healthcare system so different in terms of cost? Many of the nations whose per capita healthcare costs are half the cost of the United States' are industrialized, high-tech nations. Much of the high-tech medical equipment used in the United States is manufactured in those nations. Why are their costs so low?

The argument that higher per capita income drives higher per capita healthcare spending cannot by itself account for the differences in cost. Luxemburg has a substantially higher per capita income than the United States, but per capita healthcare costs in that nation are 40% less than in the United States. Even the next least efficient nation in terms of per capita healthcare costs, Switzerland, spends 30% less per capita on healthcare than the United States but has greater life expectancy.[5,6]

What is different in the United States than in these countries? Figure 1 plots the per capita healthcare cost relative to per capita income for several nations. In the case of the United States this reflects the cost of caring for the uninsured as well as the insured population. Take note of the cluster of industrialized nations near the center of the graph. The average per capita cost of healthcare among this group is approximately *half* the per capita cost of healthcare in the United States.[5]

One immediately evident difference is that all these nations have universal healthcare policies, meaning that all their citizens have healthcare coverage. Among industrialized nations without a universal healthcare policy, The United States stands alone. This major difference raises the question, "does universal healthcare by itself contribute to lower healthcare costs?"

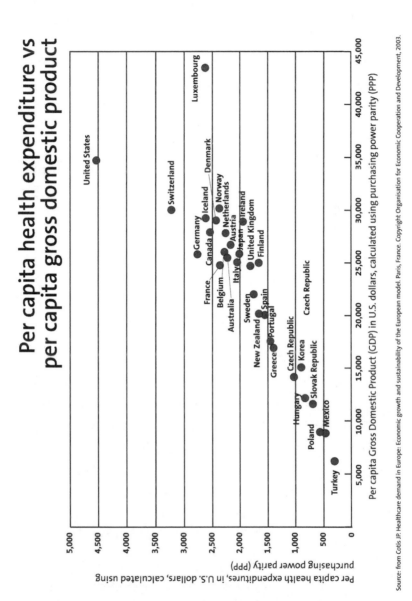

Per capita health expenditure vs per capita gross domestic product

Per capita Gross Domestic Product (GDP) in U.S. dollars, calculated using purchasing power parity (PPP)

Per capita health expenditures, in U.S. dollars, calculated using purchasing power parity (PPP)

Source: from Cotis JP. Healthcare demand in Europe: Economic growth and sustainability of the European model. Paris, France. Copyright Organisation for Economic Cooperation and Development, 2003.

Figure 1: Healthcare Cost Relative to Productivity

One immediately evident difference is that all these nations have universal healthcare policies, meaning that all their citizens have healthcare coverage. Among the industrialized nations, the United States stands alone as the only nation without a universal healthcare policy. This major difference raises the question, "does universal healthcare by itself contribute to lower healthcare costs?"

Other differences are less obvious, but built into the universal healthcare policies of many nations are explicit policy instruments that fall into three large interrelated categories: competitive market principles, consumer protections, and defined cooperative roles for both government and private insurers.

These healthcare systems have been operating for decades; the successful as well as the unsuccessful features of each system are open to review. Is there really any reason why the United States should not achieve universal healthcare and achieve lower healthcare costs? It is unconscionable that the largest economy in the world should neglect the healthcare needs of fifteen percent of its citizens and simultaneously encourage its health insurance industry to reap ever-increasing profits.

The United States Healthcare system leaks lives and dollars like a sieve. It neglects the needy and the poor. It is immoral. It is expensive. It is inefficient. It is, quite simply, broken.

CHAPTER TWO

Lofty Goals

The goal of any universal healthcare system is, in simply stated terms, to assure universal access to healthcare at a reasonable cost. Millions of Americans consider this a worthy goal. It is a goal that has not yet been achieved in the United States, but it has been achieved with remarkable success in Europe and Japan.

> It is a misconception that all European countries have single-payor healthcare systems. Some do; most do not.

Notably, it is not true that this goal has only been achieved by single-payor healthcare systems. In fact, it is a misconception that all European countries have single-payor healthcare systems. Some do; most do not. Multi-payor systems generally involve both government health insurance (GHI) and private health insurance (PHI) providers playing complementary roles, whereas single-payor systems have only a government healthcare program.

When comparing the universal healthcare systems of other countries, one soon realizes that each country has a different solution to the need for a healthcare system. Not only are these healthcare systems different from the United States' system, they are quite different even from one another. The reasons for studying these systems are, of course, to discover the successful features of other policies and to find insights that might be applicable to reform of the United States' healthcare system.

Market Failure in the Absence of Policy

The United States has a failed healthcare market. This is in no small way the consequence of a failed health insurance market.

Market failure is identified when three conditions are present:
- *increasing prices,*
- *increasing profits, and*
- *decreasing availability in the face of continued demand.*

All three identifying conditions of market failure are realized in the United States healthcare system.

It is no secret that healthcare costs consistently increase at a rate greater than the rate of inflation. Large health insurance companies continue to report increasing profits. And the United States' healthcare market certainly demonstrates decreasing availability.

Not only do forty-five million, or about fifteen percent, of Americans have no healthcare coverage; both the absolute number and percent of Americans without health coverage continue to rise. Annually about 18,000

Americans die prematurely due to lack of healthcare access.[9] These are bitter numbers; they sadden the heart. Cost adversely affected healthcare decisions for one–half of adults with health problems in the U.S. in the past year; these are patients who said they did not see a doctor when sick, did not get recommended treatment, or did not fill a prescription because of cost.[10] This deadly failure of Americans to obtain healthcare coverage confirms a failed market for both medical services and health insurance.

The United States has no healthcare policy — several agencies, but no unifying policy. Somehow, it has escaped policy makers' attention that a universal healthcare policy changes healthcare market dynamics and lowers healthcare costs. Consequently, the United States continues to pay significantly more for healthcare than industrialized nations in Europe and on the Pacific Rim.

The Organization for Economic Cooperation and Development (OECD) is one of the organizations that grew from the Marshall Plan following World War II. The OECD has thirty member nations and deals with a number of issues related to economic development, including international commerce, taxation, banking, agricultural and industrial development, and of course, healthcare. Among the industrialized nations, the United States stands alone for at least two reasons; the amount it spends on healthcare, and the proportion of its population without healthcare coverage. The United States has the most costly system in the OECD with the greatest, by far, per capita healthcare costs. Switzerland has the second most costly per capita healthcare costs and yet in 2003 spent 29% less per capita on healthcare than the United States and achieved comparable health outcome indicators. (Switzerland requires by law that all citizens enroll in a private health insurance plan.) The average per capita healthcare cost among all OECD member nations in 2003 was more than 50% less than the per capita healthcare cost in the United States. At some point, it must become apparent that universal enrollment in a healthcare plan affects healthcare markets in ways that lower overall per capita healthcare costs.

It is almost surreal that the United States cannot develop a policy for universal healthcare. Every nation in Europe has done this! Admittedly, there is no decree chiseled in stone which mandates that every nation MUST have universal healthcare, but United States citizens continue to pay in terms of both dollars and poor healthcare service for want of such a policy!

It is tempting to believe, when studying the universal healthcare policies of the various countries of the OECD, that somewhere among these systems lies some simple answer, some quick-fix solution that will mend the entire U.S. system in one stroke. Nothing could be further from reality — healthcare systems are far too complex. The successful policies of other nations have evolved over time; nations continue to measure the effectiveness of incremental changes in their healthcare policies.

Access and Solvency: Measuring the Success of Healthcare Policy

Two easily understood measures, access and solvency, reveal the effectiveness of policy and policy change, of funding strategies, manpower utilization, and the availability of infrastructure. It is true there are other measures of a healthcare system including health outcomes, but access and solvency are fundamental and are closely related. No system can sustain universal access without maintaining solvency. Access ultimately serves as a surrogate measure of solvency.

Success in addressing the issue of access will be revealed as the achievement of two conditions: 1) having nearly 100% of the population with healthcare coverage, and 2) the absence of queues, or waiting times, for elective procedures. The United States has no healthcare coverage for 15% of its population, while Canada and the United Kingdom have a notable history of prolonged waiting times for procedures. The systems of these three countries therefore fail to meet the criteria of universal access without queues.

When access and solvency are lacking, the answer is all too often thought to be more money. However, the country that spends the most money per capita on healthcare, the United States, has the worst access, has states crying for more funding for indigent care, and is no shining star when it comes to healthcare outcomes. Something other than money must therefore have an effect on both access and solvency.

The challenge, when studying other healthcare systems, is to identify features other than total spending that distinguish between systems that have successfully achieved the measures of access and solvency and those that have not. Of course healthcare systems are dynamic systems. If modifications are needed to increase access, countries change their methods; if they need more funds, they find them. If they choose to limit care, they find a way to do that, too. Somehow each successful country has evolved with a system that balances the need for access with the need for solvency.

Against this moving background one feature stands out as critical to solvency: it is the policy-assigned role of Public Health Insurance (PHI) in universal healthcare systems. Multi-payor universal healthcare systems have consistently demonstrated the capacity to achieve near 100% access and remain solvent.

The Role of Private Health Insurance in Universal Healthcare

Among countries without government ownership of the entire healthcare system, but with success at achieving both access and solvency, PHI plays a pivotal role!

This is not, however, some knee-jerk response suggesting that more PHI will solve the problems attendant to universal healthcare. The success of these nations' policies represents a sophisticated interaction between the elements of policy, PHI, and Government Health Insurance (GHI). These interactions have evolved over time. Surprisingly, these successful nations have achieved the same goal using different formats. Utilizing policy to direct the function of both GHI and PHI, multi-payor universal healthcare systems have achieved access to medical care for their populations and have done so without queues for elective procedures!

Government health insurance plays a major role in most countries. All but one OECD country uses GHI as part of its national healthcare policy. That exception is Switzerland, where, by mandate, 100% of citizens are insured with PHI. The remaining countries have some portion of citizens covered by GHI. Excluding Switzerland, the proportion ranges from 100%, which occurs in several countries, to 24.7%, which occurs in the U.S.[4]

Even in countries with government owned and managed healthcare systems, policy measures frequently employ PHI to address the issues of both access and solvency. PHI covers at least 30% of the population in over a third of OECD countries; and in many more countries PHI covers a lesser portion of the population.[4]

When assigned an appropriate role and supported by appropriate policy, PHI, in a dynamic and essential way, contributes to universal healthcare at reduced costs. More than one OECD nation with a multi-payor healthcare system has successfully coordinated government healthcare and private health insurance to achieve both access and solvency — without queues, and while assuring that care is affordable.[10,11]

> **And that, of course, is the goal – to achieve access without queues and to sustain solvency with reasonable costs.**

And that, of course, is the goal — to achieve access without queues and to sustain solvency with reasonable costs!

Although the specific details may vary among many of the OECD nations' multi-payor universal healthcare systems, these systems, whether by intent or by coincidence, employ a set of common fundamental economic and business principles relative to the role of the PHI industry. These fundamental principles are straightforward; the nations that employ these principles enjoy both access and solvency.

The OECD Taxonomy for Private Health Insurance

PHI has so many roles in so many countries that the OECD has published a report titled "Proposal for a Taxonomy of Health Insurance: OECD Study on Private Health Insurance"[12] dedicated solely to describing the types and roles of health insurance among various countries. This information is included here because the vocabulary of the insurance industry in The United States is slightly different from that used in other OECD nations.

Briefly, this report describes four major categories of PHI (*comments added within underlined parentheses*):

Primary PHI: Private insurance that represents the only available access to basic health cover when individuals do not have public (government) health insurance. This could be because there is no public health insurance, individuals are not eligible to cover under public health insurance, or they are entitled to public coverage but have chosen to opt out of such coverage. (Primary insurance covers medically necessary curative services. It is instructive, but perhaps not very important, for Americans to know that primary PHI is defined in Europe relative to the functions performed by GHI.)

Substitute: Private insurance for health costs which substitutes for cover which would otherwise be available from a social insurance (government organized plan) or publicly financed insurance (GHI) or employer's scheme (corporate self insurance). (Substitute insurance is relevant in situations where people have the opportunity, under certain conditions, to opt out of GHI.)

Principal: Private insurance for health costs, which for the insured individual represents the only available access to cover where a social security scheme (GHI) does not apply. This includes employer's compulsory schemes if cover is privately insured or self-insured.

Duplicate PHI: Private insurance that offers cover for health services already included under public health insurance. Duplicate health insurance can be marketed as an option to the public sector because, while it offers access to the same medical services as the public scheme, it also offers access to different providers or levels of service, such as: i) access to private health facilities that are not accessible through public insurance when the full cost of the service is paid by private insurance; ii) access to fast/privileged cover by bypassing queues in public system; II) access to care independent from referral and gatekeeper systems; iv) choice of doctor, hospital, or other health provider. Notably, subscribing to duplicate health insurance does not exempt individuals from contributing to public health insurance.

(There is no specific Duplicate Health Insurance market in the U.S.)

Complementary PHI: Private insurance that complements coverage provided by Primary Insurance, whether publicly insured services (GHI) or services within principal/substitute health insurance (PHI). Complementary insurance pays, either totally or in part, only toward that proportion of qualifying care costs that are not otherwise reimbursed by Primary Insurance (whether GHI or PHI). (Comparable insurance is sold in the U.S. and pays toward deductibles and co-payments; in other words, the portion of medical bills not paid by the primary insurer. An example is Medigap, which pays toward the unpaid portion of medical bills for Medicare patients.)

Supplementary PHI: Private health insurance that provides cover for additional health services not covered by either GHI or Primary PHI. Depending on the country, it may include services such as luxury care, elective care, long-term care, dental care, eye glasses, pharmaceuticals, rehabilitation, alternative or complementary medicine, etc., or superior hotel and amenity hospital services (even when other portions of the service--i.e. medical component--are covered by the primary insurer, public or private).

These OECD definitions are seldom adhered to in the U.S. When asked what "supplementary insurance" means, most Americans unwittingly change the word "supplementary" to "supplemental" and give the OECD definition for Complementary Insurance. What does that mean? Probably not much. It mostly means that Americans just don't have the inclination to sit around visiting about different kinds of health insurance.

What it means in this book is that from now on, Duplicate, Complementary or Supplementary Insurance will be mentioned only by name. The terms *insurance* or PHI will refer to a basic healthcare benefits package that covers medically necessary curative services that could be purchased from a private insurer in the U.S., whether from an HMO, a PPO, or an indemnity insurance company. In other words, basic private health insurance — PHI.

From all this conversation about the taxonomy of health insurance there is a lesson to be learned; it is that the health insurance industry is an extremely versatile business. Private health insurance thrives and is capable of providing primary, duplicate, complementary and supplementary insurance in a wide variety of regulatory situations. Even though each of the thirty OECD countries has a different system for providing healthcare coverage, the insurance industry has found a niche in most of them and, in fact, performs a vital policy role. One might therefore suppose that PHI will be perfectly capable of accepting a responsible and dynamic role in any multi-payor universal healthcare policy developed in the U.S. And when the U.S. develops its universal healthcare system, as it one day assuredly will, that system will very likely be a multi-payor system with GHI and PHI playing complementary roles, as they so commonly do in other member countries of the OECD.

℞

The remainder of this book is divided into three parts; the first part, chapters three through eight, contains background information, a description of eight different healthcare systems, and definitions of some of the terms and problems associated with the universal healthcare debate. Chapters nine through twelve suggest a model for the United States that preserves market competition, choices for clients enrolling in healthcare plans, and assures universal healthcare enrollment. This model is intended only as a starting point for further discussion. Chapter thirteen is a conclusion and review of the national benefits derived from universal healthcare.

CHAPTER THREE

Policy – What Goes In and What Comes Out

As described in the previous chapter, PHI is a versatile business, and as an adjunct to GHI, fulfills roles that GHI is not equipped to accomplish. The OECD countries with multi-payor healthcare systems frequently enlist the peculiar features of PHI when implementing healthcare policy; some countries seem to have had greater success than others in the process of integrating PHI into healthcare policy. Interestingly, there are several studies relative to the advantages and disadvantages of these different healthcare systems.[1,4,13,14,15] This chapter discusses the relationship between GHI and PHI.

> For any country to advance a universal healthcare plan, it must first develop a healthcare policy.

For any country to advance a universal healthcare plan it must first develop a healthcare policy and, in that policy, must define the roles of both GHI and PHI. It may seem obtuse to state that neither GHI nor PHI can perform tasks to which they are unsuited, but it is not quite as obvious to state what those tasks might be. The role of each has evolved over time, and the awareness of the capacity of each has likewise evolved; and in some symbiotic fashion governments have shaped policy with relationships between GHI and PHI suitable to their own needs.[1]

It is noteworthy that the Scandinavian countries have largely single-payor healthcare systems with 100% of their populations covered by state owned and managed healthcare systems. But even here there is a modest market for supplementary and a small market for complementary insurance. The culture of Scandinavian countries contributes to the success of these socialized healthcare systems; these people are not the oppressed victims of tyrannical socialist regimes — these people are socialist. Social welfare is a priority among them, and consequently they expect their governments to participate in the welfare of their lives. They pay in excess of 50% of their incomes in taxes, and they elect managers as government leaders who can accomplish their social agenda, including healthcare.

But most OECD countries are somewhat more capitalist in their philosophies, and in order to implement universal healthcare systems, government policy makers have assumed certain responsibilities for themselves and have assigned certain other roles to both GHI and PHI institutions.

First, Have a Policy.

Government must assume the role of policy maker and, relative to healthcare, must reserve certain powers to itself. Government may then assign certain responsibilities to GHI, and may allow PHI certain privileges and impose upon PHI certain constraints in order to accomplish the public goals of access and solvency for the healthcare system. As mentioned before, there is no one "right" way to assign these responsibilities and privileges, but there are some common functions that must be addressed; and both GHI and PHI must be assigned appropriate and complementary roles if any healthcare policy is to be successfully implemented.

Governments must reserve to themselves the responsibility of defining healthcare policy. They must examine available resources, allocate them, and then hope they have planned well or adapt when they have not. OECD nations have dealt with the issues of access and solvency in a variety of ways and with varying degrees of success. Some countries are able both to provide access and to remain solvent, a few countries remain solvent but have limited access, and some countries have chronic problems with both access and solvency. Because the relationship between GHI and PHI affects access and solvency, it is important to understand their roles relative to one another.

Simply announcing that everyone has access to healthcare does not assure that everyone actually has the services they need. Infrastructure is costly.

Manpower is costly. Access and solvency cannot, therefore, be separated. It must soon become apparent that not everyone will have every medical service they desire without cost. There is always a natural tension between access and solvency, and some means of limiting the consumption of medical services — some balance between access and solvency — invariably evolves. In times of economic downturn, almost every country wrestles with that balance. The need for medical services does not necessarily follow economic cycles. The ability of a country to maintain that balance requires good policy.

Advantages and Disadvantages of Government Health Insurance

Among the tools available to governments when planning the structure of a healthcare system are both GHI and PHI. They may choose either or both as instruments of policy. When governments accept the responsibility of providing universal healthcare, or more correctly, *are assigned that responsibility by their people,* there are certain additional policy roles that government must also accept. These include:

- *Government protects vulnerable populations; government defines those populations and makes accommodation for them. (PHI, left without other direction, will not adopt this task.)*

- *Government defines the level of healthcare benefits and thus assures a certain "level of care" (usually determined through legislation); government may exclude or include risky or experimental or unproven services at its discretion.*

- *Government assures the equitable distribution of services; it is counter productive to promise universal healthcare and then discriminate in the distribution of care.*

- *Government addresses public health concerns in a way that complements its other responsibilities; without a Public Health policy attentive to disease prevention there is increased potential for costly epidemics. (In the present United States system GHI inherits the consequences of Public Health policy when the population reaches age 65.)*

The disadvantages of government health programs include:

- *The government revenue stream is fixed by tax revenues. GHI is dependent upon taxation to fund all its services and must operate within the budget defined by those revenues.*

- *Government may implement only those services and technologies for which funds are available.*

- *Fees for services may be set in order to contain costs.*

    - *This limits cash flow and the funding of new infrastructure.*

    - *This discourages providers from seeing patients for which payment is fixed at a low rate.*

- *There is a disconnect between the revenue stream and the demand for medical services.*

    - *The revenue stream is determined by the willingness of the electorate to be taxed.*

    - *The demand for medical services has nothing to do with the willingness of the electorate to be taxed but is instead dependent upon the prevalence of disease.*

    - *The demand for medical services does not necessarily follow economic cycles.*

- *There is a disconnect between the revenue stream and the determination of benefits.*

- *In Canada the federal government retains control of benefits, but the provinces are mandated to provide the financing.*

- *In the United States' Medicaid program there is a mandate to states to provide care for the very poor, but insufficient federal funding to do so.*

Advantages and Disadvantages of Private Health Insurance

PHI fulfills a somewhat different set of functions than government, and there are differing opinions as to its relative merits. Reviewers of government policy regarding health insurance note that PHI has the following advantages and disadvantages.

Recognized advantages to a government that includes PHI in healthcare policy are:

- *PHI is a financing and payment mechanism for healthcare services.*

- *Cash flowing through PHI provides a source of funding for infrastructure, technology and research.*

- *PHI is more sensitive to market demands (patient utilization patterns) than GHI.*

- *PHI relieves GHI of certain costs and caseloads.*

- *PHI rewards innovation and efficiency (in its own industry).*

- *PHI must remain solvent (without raising taxes).*

- *PHI limits utilization and enhances personal accountability, at least to an extent tolerable to the healthcare market, through the use of deductibles and co-pays.*[4,13]

The capacity of PHI to fund infrastructure and remain solvent without relying on taxation is noteworthy.

Because PHI companies remain solvent by acquiring and retaining paying clients, and because clients may shop based on service as well as on price, PHI must support patients in obtaining the medical services they desire and must do so at a reasonable price, or clients will go elsewhere for their insurance. When clients visit doctors and hospitals and purchase elective services, they expect their insurance companies to pay the agreed upon share of medical charges. Insurance companies will do this to the extent that they are legally bound to do so and in order to maintain a content clientele. In this manner, competition for clients drives PHI to pay for elective medical services and supports a market for medical care. It is from the simple necessity of remaining solvent that PHI promotes a market for healthcare services and gathers funds to pay for the infrastructure required to perform those services, whether these are basic services, elective services, or supplementary services.[4,13]

PHI has some important disadvantages. Left to compete based on risk, PHI will price-discriminate, pricing coverage out of the reach of patients with increased health risk or pre-existing illness, (and perhaps someday refusing to insure patients with certain genetic markers). Those with the greatest need for medical care will not have medical care available.

Left to compete on the basis of administrative costs, PHI will once again price-discriminate and charge higher fees to small businesses and to individual insurees. Those with the least bargaining power will pay the highest premiums. In a variation on this theme, in situations where buyers have limited negotiating power, they may have lower premium costs but greater out-of-pocket costs in the form of deductibles and co-pays and be left with higher total healthcare costs.[40,41]

Unless regulated to perform otherwise, PHI favors elective procedures; physicians are more likely to perform an elective procedure or a diagnostic test for a patient paying full price through PHI than for a patient paying a limited fee with GHI.

In summary PHI has the following disadvantages:

- *PHI is inclined to provide services preferentially to the healthy and the wealthy.*

- *PHI excludes clients with the greatest health risks.*[4]

- *PHI tends to direct resources toward elective services.*

Both GHI and PHI promote over-utilization.[4] Notably, several OECD nations have successfully implemented regulations that address these disadvantages specifically, as will be discussed in subsequent chapters.

Advantages of Using Both Government and Private Insurers to Provide Primary Care

The combined utilization of both GHI and PHI has this particular advantage: when PHI collects and redistributes monies that eventually fund medical infrastructure, then, once that infrastructure is in place, GHI clients may use it at or near marginal cost! An example of this is when CT scanners first became available in the U.S. Medicare in the U.S. was reluctant to pay for the use of this expensive new technology, but physicians loved the additional information they got from CT scans and ordered them for their Medicare patients anyway. Medicare patients thus gained access to valuable new technology even though GHI had been reluctant to contribute to its funding. GHI soon paid for CT scans, but at a fee below what private insurers pay.

Private insurees also benefit from this arrangement. The more frequently any technology is used, the lower the marginal costs become for all users.

Conclusion

Neither GHI nor PHI has the capacity to perform in the manner that the other performs. There are disadvantages to government-managed systems that have been demonstrated by other nations and that should not be repeated.

(For example, a recent pair of court decisions overturned the long-standing monopoly of the Canadian federal government as the single healthcare payor in that country, opening the door to having primary insurance through private insurers.[16,17] "Access to a waiting list is not access to health care," according to Chief Justice Beverley McLachlin.)

It has been an important lesson for policy makers that healthcare spending channeled through PHI reflects the critical healthcare services patients

> "Access to a waiting list is not access to health care." The Right Honourable Beverley McLachlin, P.C., Chief Justice of Canada.

need and use. This channeling of resources also reveals preferences regarding elective services. Through PHI mechanisms, the infrastructure for those services is financed, and once the infrastructure is in place, patients with GHI have access to that infrastructure.

GHI would seem content to spend no more than it must on medical infrastructure, and would prefer to pay only for basic services. This is intuitively understandable; in order to provide additional infrastructure and deliver a wider selection of elective services, GHI must resort to taxation for additional revenues (seldom popular). PHI, on the other hand, simply does the accounting and adjusts premiums in response to patients' demands for services. PHI, after all, promotes a market for medical services, and success in any market means providing for customers the goods and services for which they will pay.

Again, the private health insurance industry behaves differently than government healthcare; neither of the two sectors, government or private, functions perfectly. Each has weaknesses; each has advantages. Nations that have minimized the disadvantages and maximized the advantages have universal healthcare, excellent outcomes measures, and have no waiting times for elective procedures.

Every system and every tool has constraints. Certainly, if government intends to develop a healthcare policy, *and* recognizes the weakness of single-payor systems, *and* wishes to employ the advantages of PHI as a policy tool, then government must accommodate both the advantages and disadvantages of *both* PHI and GHI; but it will harvest the advantage of having infrastructure available to meet patient demands.

CHAPTER FOUR

A Variety of Models

Access is invariably a reflection of solvency. If resources are not available, someone must go without timely access to care. The phenomenon of limiting the delivery of medical services by restricting resources is referred to as "soft rationing." One measure of soft rationing is prolonged waiting times for elective procedures. With this in mind, it is worth reviewing the organizational structures of a few of the healthcare systems of OECD countries, paying particular attention to what percentage of the population has true access and whether observed waiting times for elective procedures are prolonged.

For the U.S., 85% of the population has real access to all medical services, and there is no observed waiting time for those with access. (Of course, for those without access, for elective procedures and even for some life preserving procedures, waiting times may be infinite.) For some nations, soft rationing is the acknowledged method of maintaining solvency.

There is one additional question to be asked about solvency: How does the system meet the costs of growth in the healthcare industry?

This is a question that deals not with the immediate methods of funding, but with measures to accommodate growth of the healthcare industry in general. New technologies make it possible to live longer, healthier lives; and when people use those technologies, it is only natural that the industry will grow. We consider growth in most industries to be beneficial, yet governments, under budget constraints to limit healthcare spending, retain a tendency to contain growth in the healthcare industry.[18] But devoting more of GDP to healthcare as society gets richer is not necessarily inappropriate.[19]

Solvency must address not only current access, but also growth in the healthcare industry and economic cycles. As we review a few countries' healthcare systems, we will see that economic cycles disrupt tax-based funding mechanisms when there is an economic downturn.

Case Studies

The following case studies provide examples of the different methods of organizing universal healthcare systems among the member nations of the OECD. There are important contrasts between these countries' systems. Each system is unique. Some of the systems were initially intended to completely socialize healthcare; most were not. All have gone through a process of slow evolution to meet the demands of social and economic change.

Canada

In 1957 Canada instituted the Canadian insurance system and passed the Hospital Insurance Act, which provided for federal and provincial governments to share the costs of hospitalization on an equal basis (50-50). All provinces were organized under a national universal healthcare system by 1961, under which the management and delivery of healthcare services were the responsibility of the provinces and territories, and the national healthcare agenda was set at the federal level.

The system has undergone several revisions over time, changing the methods of transferring funds from the federal government to the provinces. In 1977 Canada passed the Program Funding Act. This act linked medical funding to educational funding. Federal contributions to healthcare benefits also dropped from 50% to 29%. In 1984 the Canada Health Act replaced previous legislation and further reduced federal payments, placing the responsibility for funding more heavily on the provinces. The federal contribution to funding is now at 15%. The definition of coverage has been modified to include "medically necessary services" and some coverage for drugs, medical devices and home care. The effect is that services are now rationed based on "medical necessity," and there are waiting lists for many services –

the management of which is a perennial topic for Canadian healthcare managers.[20-22]

The federal government maintains its commitment to set national criteria for healthcare services, including universal portability, while placing the responsibility for funding on the provinces. Costs to the provinces have continued to rise, personal healthcare spending has continued to rise, and debate continues over healthcare funding. Oil-rich Alberta is the only province able to fund its healthcare services without heavily shifting costs to patients. Canadians acknowledge that provider incentives are related to volume, not to outcomes, and that there is redundancy and duplication in its administrative system. Fiscal restraints limit development of new infrastructure, training of providers, and the introduction of new technology; specialized services are available only in metropolitan areas. Thus access is assured by federal mandate, promoting moral hazard, but services are rationed at the provincial level due to lack of facilities and manpower,[23] and waiting times for medical services are observed to be prolonged relative to other OECD countries.[4] The results are soft rationing of medical care, and a *de facto* tiered system with the wealthy going out-of-country for elective medical services.

United Kingdom

The United Kingdom initiated single payor universal healthcare in 1948 with the creation of the National Health Service (NHS). The NHS differs from most public healthcare systems in Continental Europe; it not only pays for healthcare expenses, it also employs the doctors and nurses that provide them, and runs hospitals and clinics. In the immediate period following WWII, attitudes and expectations toward social programs were optimistic. Services were provided entirely free of charge at the point of use and were financed from central taxation. Everyone was eligible for care, even people temporarily resident or visiting the country. Reality had to be confronted very soon, and by 1952 spiraling costs led to the introduction of a charge for prescriptions, and also a charge for dental treatment. Through the 1970s and 1980s, it became increasingly clear that the NHS would never have the resources necessary to provide unlimited access to the latest medical treatments.[24]

The NHS continues to provide good services and basic care, but lack of capacity — facilities and personnel — results in soft rationing.[4] Waiting times have become a chronic complaint with the NHS, where waiting lists are now an ongoing topic of study.[25-29] The proposed solutions to this problem are to increase infrastructure and financial incentives.[30] Preliminary evidence also suggests that an increase in private health insurance coverage may reduce waiting times.[30]

Although a small, privately-funded healthcare system has always existed alongside the NHS, the vast majority of Britons get their healthcare through the publicly funded NHS.

Debate about how providers are paid persists in the UK. In the 1990s, the NHS introduced an "internal market" into its system hoping to promote competition and reduce costs. A system of provider contracts was established wherein physicians are not remunerated directly for the services they provide; rather, general practitioners are paid for maintaining the health of populations for whom they are responsible. To share risk and improve management efficiencies, physician groups have combined the contracts or "funds" from which they are paid. This system has been difficult to manage; money does not "follow the patient," meaning that providers are not necessarily paid depending on either the complexity of the work they do or on the amount. This has resulted in a tiered system favoring persons requiring less complicated — and less expensive — procedures, and "funded" patients, and has not resulted in diminished waiting times. [4,24] Furthermore, this new system has not introduced any real competition. Efficient providers have not been allowed to retain the profits of their efficiency, and inefficient providers have not necessarily been penalized for their inefficiency.[4]

Greengross, Grant, et al. stated in 1999 in the closing paragraph of *The History and Development of the UK National Health Service*:

> It is inevitable that, in the face of limited resources, rather than expecting the NHS to provide everyone with all forms of care, healthcare will need to be rationed and a consensus achieved as to what the service's aims should be in the 21st Century.[24]

The Netherlands

Universal healthcare in the Netherlands has been achieved through a combination of GHI and PHI; roughly two-thirds of the population, 64%, are covered by GHI, and just less than one third, 31%, are covered by PHI. The remaining 5%, mostly civil servants, are covered by a special GHI fund, and a small fraction of chronically debilitated patients are covered under the Exceptional Medical Expenses Act. The roughly one third covered by PHI are the wealthiest segment of the population. These are considered to be the most capable members of society and the least dependent upon receiving healthcare through GHI; they are therefore mandated to purchase PHI. By regulation, insurers must allow any applicant to purchase insurance (guaranteed issue), and insurers may not price differentiate based on risk (community rating).[4]

To assure that clients of PHI do not receive preferential medical treatment, PHI and GHI, by regulation, must reimburse for services at the same rate — a rate set by GHI — and patients under either PHI or GHI receive similar services and treatments regardless of insurance status.

Eighty-five percent of GHI is paid for with worker and employee contributions based on income level; the balance is paid from revenues from a national consumption tax. PHI is purchased either through employment, at a rate of about 60%, or independently.[4]

The Netherlands is one of the OECD countries that intentionally fosters PHI as a policy measure, believing that a mixed private/public health system can better deliver health services and social outcomes. PHI contributes funding to healthcare services in ways that GHI does not, and that PHI is a source of funding for healthcare infrastructure independent from tax revenues, thus generating increased capacity in the healthcare system. PHI also brings sensitivity to the market for healthcare services and increased choice among services.[4,12,13]

Until recently, the Netherlands has had no observed waiting times for elective procedures. The global economic downturn of the early twenty-first century affected the Netherlands, along with other countries, spurring a desire in that country to implement a "self sustaining" healthcare system. Other factors contributed to this desire, including an aging population, an inadequate public health policy (the Netherlands has done little to curb the use of tobacco or other practices harmful to health), supply side controls (fee setting), and an acknowledged disconnect between revenue streams for GHI and the payment for GHI services.

This disconnect occurs because the public system is based on the "Solidarity system." The Solidarity system is based on the rather socially attractive concept that each should pay according to their capacity and receive according to their needs. In reality this means that worker-employer contributions to healthcare are based on the workers' wages, but there is not necessarily a correlation between the productivity (wages) of employees and the need for healthcare services. In times of economic downturn, the need for healthcare services may outpace wages and therefore healthcare revenues.

Features of the new, self-regulating healthcare system include many existing policies as well as some changed policies as follows:

- *Participation in health insurance, either GHI or PHI, is mandatory.*

- *Any distinctions between services obtained through PHI or GHI must be abolished.*

- *Insurers may not differentiate premiums or out-of-pocket expenses for insurees.*

- *Every adult contributes an out-of-pocket amount toward a uniform, broad basic package of healthcare benefits with a compulsory deductible.*

- *An income-independent employer contribution allows revenues from client contributions to be more sensitive to the use of healthcare services.*

- *Lower income individuals are to be compensated from a new health fund.*

- *Public health policy is to be reviewed and enhanced.*

- *Health insurers will negotiate with providers regarding the price of medical services.*

Policy makers have adopted an evidence-based approach in making these decisions, pragmatism being the guiding principle.

France

The French, in the spirit of égalité, have elected to provide GHI for 100% of the population, but only for a portion of healthcare expenses. GHI pays approximately 72% for physician services, up to 100% for critical medications, but as low as 65% for "convenience medications" and up to 92% for hospital services. GHI is financed by a national consumption tax, as are most social services.

Private insurance existed in France long before government involvement in healthcare. PHI takes various forms; about 60% are non-profit "mutuelles" (Couverture Mutuelle Universal — CMU). About 40% are private insurance companies; about half of these are for-profit and half are not-for-profit companies. Private insurance, in its various forms, now provides complementary insurance to 86% of the population; the government subsidizes another 6% of the population with complementary insurance so that 100% of the population has basic coverage through GHI and 92% of the population has complementary insurance. Much of the population also purchases supplementary insurance. This combination of GHI and PHI ultimately pays for about 88% of total healthcare expenditures; the balance is out-of-pocket expense.

PHI is used by policy makers in France much the same way it is in the Netherlands — as an additional source of revenue to increase the capacity of the healthcare system, and as a means of enhancing market responsiveness and increasing consumer choice. PHI also assumes the role of containing over-utilization. France has not been immune to the financial problems generated by downturns in economic cycles and certain proponents advocate further reforms.

Switzerland

Switzerland has had a national healthcare policy since 1911. The policy underwent revisions in 1996. There is no GHI in Switzerland; by mandate 100% of the population is to be covered by PHI (actually about 1% has no coverage). A uniform policy is offered by all providers, prompting insurers to compete on price and service. Eighty percent of the population has some form of complementary or supplementary insurance. For basic insurance coverage, insurers may not differentiate price or co-payments based on risk or deny coverage based on pre-existing conditions or health status. Cost allowances are made for children and students. Price differentiation is allowed for supplementary insurance. Insurers, by mandate, participate in a reinsurance program referred to as a "risk-redistribution" system which serves to equalize the risk to insurers who accept high risk populations.

In this setting, PHI defines the entire market for health insurance and is the funding mechanism for most healthcare services. The government, primarily at the local level, directs and subsidizes the construction of hospitals and also subsidizes individuals in need of financial assistance.

The government has built an environment where, in order to promote competition, there are several competing PHI providers. Although switching insurers is allowed during specified time periods, there is relatively little switching between insurers because insurers have been allowed to bundle complementary and supplementary benefits with basic benefits with lower premiums for bundled packages. Clients are reluctant to switch to insurers with lower basic rates for fear of losing or paying higher rates for complementary or supplementary insurance.

To the degree that these barriers to switching between insurers impede market competition, insurers are able to charge somewhat higher prices for healthcare coverage.

The healthcare infrastructure has adequate capacity, and there are no observed waiting times for elective procedures. Over-utilization is managed with deductibles and co-pays, and providers are paid for the services they provide — money follows the patient. About a third of total health expenditures in Switzerland are out-of-pocket.[4]

Ireland

The Irish healthcare system continues to evolve. The most recent changes have taken place in the private sector and have been directed by the courts. The most recent developments reaffirm the desire of the Irish government to share some of the responsibility for the nation's healthcare burden with the private sector in a market environment.

As early as 1957, the public system provided free access to hospital services to lower and middle income individuals. The wealthiest 15% of the population was excluded from public coverage and was expected to purchase its own healthcare.

In 1957, Ireland also passed the Voluntary Health Insurance Act. This act established the Voluntary Health Insurance Board, now known as the VHI, a not-for-profit government sponsored entity (a statutory corporation with legal status similar to the Public Broadcasting System in the U.S.) that provided, and still provides, the equivalent of "private" health insurance.

The VHI had a monopoly-like status over the private health insurance industry until, in 1994, in response to a directive of the Council of European Communities, Ireland passed the Health Insurance act of 1994 and invited other private health insurance companies into its market. Consequently, the Irish healthcare market is now divided between the public sector (about 51% of the population), the VHI (about 39%), and competitive private health insurance companies (about 10% of the population.) Individuals are given a tax benefit for enrolling with either the VHI or a private health insurance company. Forty-nine percent of the population takes advantage of this and leave the public plan favoring a private plan or its near equivalent, the VHI.

Among the policies enacted for the VHI in 1957 were community rating, lifetime cover, and open enrollment ("lifetime cover" and "open enrollment" being the equivalent of "guaranteed issue.") Then in 1979, the remaining 15% of the population was granted publicly funded hospital enrollment. This was enacted as a default enrollment policy so that now the population had universal coverage for hospitalization.

The 1994 act had opened the market to private insurers and retained the policies for lifetime cover and open enrollment. In 1996, Insurance Regulations based on the 1994 act added regulations for standard minimum benefits. (Whether this was enacted as the political response to pressures for "social justice" or for humanitarian reasons or for economic reasons I do not know, but this much is apparent: the Irish now had a system with universal enrollment (on a default basis), community ratings, guaranteed issue and minimum benefits.)

The 1996 Insurance Regulations also provided for a "risk-equalization" plan, essentially a reinsurance plan to distribute risk across the entire population. When The British United Provident Association (BUPA) started doing business in Ireland in 1997 the company marketed to younger healthier populations – practicing what is commonly referred to as "cherry picking." BUPA later declined to pay the fees that VHI claimed it owed under the risk-equalization plan. The Supreme Court decided in late 2006 that BUPA owed the fees. BUPA announced it would quit doing business in Ireland and sold its business in Ireland to the Quinn Group in January 2007. (BUPA is an international insurer with revenues in 2004 of over GBP 3.6 Billion.)

Thus, Ireland preserves a national healthcare system with universal (default) enrollment, community ratings, guaranteed issue and minimum benefits.

It also preserves its risk redistribution plan; all this while preserving a system where clients may chose either default enrollment in a public plan or open enrollment in a selection of private health coverage plans. Per capita healthcare costs in Ireland were US$1,900 in 2002 compared to the US costs of $4,500.

Germany

Health insurance in Germany is mandatory, and about 90% of the population is enrolled in GHI which consists of 1,200+ highly regulated, geographically organized, "sickness funds." These funds are independently managed but offer uniform health insurance benefits. No one is denied coverage; age-based community ratings assure that persons within a given age range receive coverage at a similar price regardless of health status. But because premiums are based on the client's age at enrollment, switching between funds is not common because a client switching to a different sickness fund would have to pay higher premiums based on an older age category. Caps on premiums limit the expense of insurance for the elderly and distribute risk more evenly over the entire population. A national reserve fund compensates sickness funds that accept high-risk clients.

Only the wealthy are allowed to "opt-out" of GHI, and just less than 10% of the population purchases PHI. Those who do opt out are treated at the same hospitals but may have different doctors, obtain different amenities, and may have *very* short waiting times for elective procedures.

Contributions to the state regulated sickness funds are equivalent to about 14% of a worker's gross income. This amount is shared equally by the employer and the employee. Funding for GHI is thus based on the

Solidarity concept — as it is in the Netherlands and a few other OECD countries — from each according to his ability, to each according to his need. But, as mentioned previously, this means that the revenue stream is not sensitive to the demand for medical services.

Primary GHI covers up to 68% of healthcare costs. Fees paid to the providers of GHI-funded services are set by GHI, but fees paid to the providers of PHI clients may be higher. This allows PHI clients to choose from among the most reputable providers; PHI may pay providers twice what GHI pays. This has generated an overtly tiered healthcare system, which is disconcerting to some who seek its reform.

PHI is intended as a source of additional healthcare funds and a means of reducing caseloads for GHI-provided services. Although only 10% of the population has PHI, PHI provides about 13% of total healthcare expenditures.

There is no increase in waiting times for elective procedures relative to other OECD countries.

As in the Netherlands, an aging population coupled with an economic downturn has placed financial pressure on the German healthcare system and prompted revision efforts. Policy makers recognize that a fixed healthcare budget based on revenues generated using the Solidarity system will not necessarily meet healthcare demands. There have been attempts to introduce increased competition into the system and thereby lower costs, but success in this effort has been limited. Geographic segmentation of markets limits competition, strong hospital and physician associations limit efforts at negotiations, and the nature of age-related pricing of premiums has inhibited clients from seeking lower priced insurers. There is also a conflicted attitude toward PHI; GHI would like to have the income-related revenues from this segment of the population but acknowledges the value of PHI as a market force.[4,31,32]

Japan

Japan has had many successes in its management of healthcare. Japan approaches 100% healthcare coverage. It has a vigorous public health and preventive medicine program, the greatest longevity of any country, and spends only 7.8% of GDP on healthcare.

In spite of this, there are calls for revision regarding inequities in access and the expenses associated with caring for an aging population.[4] More intensive control of prices and even volume through changes in the fee schedule, plus increases in various co-payment rates, led to an actual reduction in medical spending for the first time in 2002.[33]

Healthcare coverage is mandatory in Japan. Insurance plans fall into two large general categories; a third small category (the Health Program for the Elderly), is funded by contributions from the other two programs.

The first and largest of the general categories consists of several cooperative employee health insurance plans, of which there are three main types:

- *Shaho -- insurance cooperatives for the employees of large corporations (There are in excess of 1,800 of these highly regulated non-profit cooperatives.)*

- *Government-managed health insurance plans for employees of small businesses, of which there are over 3,000*
- *Mutual Aid Associations which provide coverage for public employees, teachers, etc.*

The costs of insurance for all employee cooperative insurance programs are shared equally between employees and employers.[34]

The second large category is Kokuho, which is the single large GHI program in Japan. Kokuho was originally set up to provide healthcare services to the agricultural sector in Japan, which, when GHI was organized in 1961, was considered a strategically important segment of the population. Kokuho now covers not only the agricultural sector, but also the self employed, their dependents and all those formerly covered by Kokuho. Kokuho is funded 50% by worker contributions and 50% by taxation.[34]

Information about healthcare costs is very transparent and fees for medical services are set following negotiations with providers based on this open knowledge of costs. Funds to pay for anticipated costs are then collected by the organizations described above. Healthcare capacity is sufficient that there are no observed waiting times for elective procedures.

Conclusion

There are thirty OECD member countries. The healthcare systems of only eight have been discussed, but even from this limited review one can see the wide variety of models of universal healthcare systems and understand that there is no one "right" model. Each model is more or less dynamic, although changes in individual national models have been observed to be slow and incremental.[1] Each has come to a balance between access and solvency. There are different policy-assigned roles for PHI in each of these countries. In each model there is a different response to the tension between access and solvency.

The relationship between the proportion of the population with PHI and access to care without waiting times is real. Among the countries reviewed, those with no waiting times have a substantial proportion of the population covered by PHI. Review of these countries' healthcare systems draws into relief the peculiar capacities of PHI. This is not to say that single-payor systems cannot or do not provide adequate healthcare, but PHI can, and in many cases does, have a significant effect on the timely delivery of medical services — on both access and solvency.

Selvoy M. Fillerup, MD, MSPH, FACS

CHAPTER FIVE

Balance, Balance, Balance

Balance is everything in the delivery of healthcare. The problem is that this balance must be multi-dimensional. It is not as simple as finding a balance between supply and demand, or between access and solvency, or between under-utilization and over-utilization of medical services, or between expenditures for public health and expenditures for tertiary care, or between pharmaceutical and hospital expenditures. Balance in healthcare requires a simultaneous balance of all these elements — and always with a balanced budget.

As shown in the previous chapter, balance between the relative advantages and disadvantages of both PHI and GHI is critical, but attainable.

Aggregate balance is achievable if the correct incentives are in place to reward individual choice. Evidence for this is all around us in competitive market societies; go look at a strip-mall, or the avenue in your town where several auto dealerships are lined up in a row, or a street lined with fast food restaurants; or read the ads in a newspaper; or follow the stock market. Aggregate balance evolves when individual choices are rewarded. This is also true when healthcare choices are made.

From another perspective, there is a tension between management goals in healthcare. On one hand, the delivery of medical services is a business; one goal must always be financial stability. This requires resources, manpower, and a balanced budget, as well as sufficient financial rewards to attract well-educated doctors, nurses, technicians, and managers, and investments in the seemingly never ending fountain of technological advances.

> On the one hand, the delivery of medical services is a business; one goal must always be financial stability. On the other hand, healthcare is a humanitarian service; its other goal is not profit, but health.

On the other hand, healthcare is a humanitarian service; its other goal is not profit, but health. Integrating these divergent goals into a single system has never been simple; measuring money is much easier than measuring health. Still, health-related goals cannot be achieved in the absence of successful business related goals.

True balance in healthcare must <u>also provide for a more subtle balance between over-utilization and under-utilization of medical services</u>. When services are too readily available, moral hazard contributes to the over-utilization of services. This not only causes unnecessary expense, but may also be harmful to health (one historic example being the inappropriate use of x-ray treatments for acne in decades past). There are also several opportunities for under-utilization of medical services. This occurs when an elective surgery is postponed for so long that irreversible debility or death results, as may be the case with orthopedic problems, heart disease or cancer.[35-38]

Whether the appropriate balance between under- and over-utilization is ever achieved will always depend on how one measures the relationship between utilization and health, and upon how one measures health. The same holds true for the relationship between the access/ solvency issue and health. Since it is policy that ultimately affects both access and solvency, it is important to remember that certain policy features will have more favorable effects on access and solvency, and therefore upon health.

Favorable Policy Instruments

Features of national health policies regarding PHI that are favorable to access and solvency include:

- *Uniformity of benefits (When countries have mandated that insurers offer a uniform basic benefits package, insurees are able to shop based on price, convenience, reputation and so on, rather than attempting to choose between dissimilar insurance products.)*

- *Large numbers of PHI providers, thus promoting a competitive market*

- *Absence of barriers to switching between providers (Specifically, we have seen how an age related rating system has hampered efforts in Germany to introduce a price competitive environment. Risk ratings in general hamper the ability to switch carriers and thus limit competition between providers. In Switzerland we observed that the bundling of basic coverage with complementary or supplementary coverage has limited the ability of insurees to change insurers. In contrast, the Netherlands has paid particular attention to regulations that preserve an environment where insurees have a broad and open choice among PHI providers.)*

• *Community ratings (Both Switzerland and the Netherlands have mandated community ratings as well as uniformity of product so that insurees may make informed choices based on price; this has kept the price of health insurance competitive.)*

• *Subsidy of vulnerable populations. (Several methods have been used to identify and provide care for the poor or the chronically ill. In the U.S. vulnerable populations have been determined to be the very poor and those over age 65. Different criteria have been set in different countries.)*

• *Demand-side price controls (Japan has accomplished this through negotiations between non-profit insurers and providers in a very transparent financial environment-- everyone knows what it costs to provide the care needed. Switzerland has accomplished this by mandating that all insurance be PHI in a competitive setting. Both these methods contribute to the solvency of their respective systems.)*

• *Guaranteed issue (This refers to the practice of issuing a policy to everyone, and anyone, who is willing to pay the price of that policy, whether they are a member of a large group or not, and regardless of their health status. If it is mandatory for all segments of the population to purchase health insurance, it only makes sense that any willing buyer may actually buy insurance at its offered price, and that there be no price differentiation--no one may be intentionally priced out of the market.)*

Unfavorable Policy Instruments

There are also some common policy features among countries that have been less favorable to the achievement of access and solvency. These are:

- *Supply-side controls (When fees are set by the government, or when money follows the system rather than the patient, there follows a shortage of manpower and infrastructure; providers are less responsive to market demands, and waiting lists reflect soft rationing and possibly unhealthy under-utilization of medical services.)*

- *A disconnect between the revenue stream and the determination of benefits (This has occurred in Canada where the federal government retains control of benefits but the provinces are mandated to provide the financing, or in the case of the United States Medicaid program, where there is a mandate to states to provide care for the very poor but insufficient federal funding to do so.)*

- *A disconnect between the revenue stream and the demand for medical services (Healthcare in both Germany and the Netherlands is financed based on the Solidarity philosophy, but during times of economic downturn there is not necessarily revenue to meet the demand for healthcare services using this method of financing.)*

- *A high proportion of the population covered by GHI (This results in attempts by GHI to contain healthcare usage and to set artificially low fees as an alternative to taxation. Canada and the United Kingdom have single-payor plans with limited participation in PHI; both have longer than average waiting lists for elective procedures; both have shortages of manpower and infrastructure.)*

- *Limited public health policy (A failure to support preventive medical practices eventually results in costs associated with chronic disease.)*

- *Narrow geographic segmentation of the market (In Germany, under conditions where markets are geographically limited and local provider associations have control over fee negotiations, there is limited competition among providers and higher costs for services.)*

Discussion

Twenty-nine of thirty OECD countries have universal healthcare; there seems to be no "right" model, but those countries without prolonged waiting times for elective procedures may be presumed to have policies that are better suited to deal with issues of solvency.

.Both GHI and PHI provide mechanisms for collecting and redistributing healthcare funds, but the mechanisms are vastly different both for collection and redistribution. GHI collects revenues either through taxation or through mandatory payroll participation, which is not dissimilar from taxation. When patient usage increases, government must assess the need for increased revenues and then muster the political will to mandate change. A lot of consensus building is required — a lot of political "mass" must be moved — to meet the changing financial needs of GHI. PHI, on the other hand, simply raises premiums in response to use patterns of patients.

GHI is almost obligated to redistribute funds within a set of parameters that are quite different from those of PHI. GHI knows, or may estimate, its revenues for the near future, but then is obligated to limit expenditures to match its revenue stream. This may mean limiting services or limiting investments in infrastructure; or, if the demand for medical services becomes too great, GHI must shift costs to other payors, either overtly to patients through co-payments, or indirectly to the clients of PHI through cost-shifting. Cost-shifting in this form is well recognized, but as budgets become tighter, and as more uniform accounting methods make costs more transparent, the PHI industry is less inclined to tolerate this practice.

GHI may contain costs by setting fees, but this generates a disinclination for some providers to accept GHI patients. A tiered system has already evolved in Germany where GHI fees are low and PHI fees are high; serious regulations have been implemented to avoid that situation in the Netherlands.

Both co-payments and fee setting affect the poor.[39] Co-payments directly dissuade the poor from seeking medical care, and fee setting acts as a disincentive for providers to accept the poor as patients. Either way, the poor are thus inclined to under-utilize primary care or preventive medical services. These measures provide incentives for the poor to wait until they must seek medical attention, a time when they are inclined to use the most expensive care available — the ER.

A lack of investment in infrastructure affects all but the wealthiest patients. Waiting lists may be economically necessary when GHI lacks funding, but the health consequences, and therefore indirect costs of delayed care, are not insignificant; waiting lists are associated with increased morbidity and mortality. The wealthy can always go elsewhere for their healthcare.

PHI, on the other hand, responds to market demands for healthcare services in a way that GHI is simply not equipped to do. PHI collects and redistributes funds for medical infrastructure in order to meet patient usage patterns. Then, once that infrastructure is in place, GHI clients may use it at or near marginal cost. PHI accepts caseloads that GHI may not be prepared to accept. PHI rewards the efficient management of its own industry. PHI increases the use of preventive care.

There is broad variety among universal healthcare models: Some are single-payor models, while others are multi-payor models employing PHI as an instrument of healthcare policy.

The issues of access and solvency confront the designers of any universal healthcare policy. When a substantial portion of the population has coverage through PHI, market economies such as those reviewed here have lower observed waiting times for elective procedures, reflecting an infrastructure and manpower supply matched to the market demands for medical services.

In the absence of regulation to direct market forces, PHI drifts toward a position of price discrimination based on risk and administrative costs and ultimately a tiered healthcare system biased against the poor and unhealthy.[11,40,41] When regulations are in place to assure access to PHI (mandatory enrollment and guaranteed issue for all applicants) and to prevent price discrimination (community ratings), PHI fulfills a valuable role generating a source of funding for healthcare infrastructure, promoting market sensitivity and a market for the use of medical services, and assuring solvency by the very nature of private enterprise to remain profitable in competitive markets.

The U.S. already has in place many of the necessary elements for a successful multi-payor universal healthcare system: GHI has defined vulnerable populations; a competitive infrastructure including hospitals, clinics, universities, and research centers is in place with strong management tools; and a large portion of the population has PHI.

But the foundation has yet to be laid — there is, as yet, no policy stating that there shall be a universal healthcare system in the United States. And without that policy in place, there are no defined roles for either GHI or PHI. In particular, there are no regulations to improve the way PHI participates relative to policy objectives. In spite of the many favorable features already in place, without a unifying policy, and without a defined role, PHI is left to act in its own best interest — but not always in the best interests of all parties.

A chicken-and-egg relationship exists between a plan and a policy; it is hard to know which really comes first. Perhaps a better analogy is the relationship between a building and its foundation: no one builds a foundation without some idea of what the building will look like, and no one plans a building without knowing what the foundation will sustain. Back to healthcare — which will come first, a viable plan or a comprehensive policy?

Circumstance has placed the United States in a position to examine the plans and policy experiences that have already occurred among other OECD member countries. The successes and failures of policy and the relative successes of the various assigned roles for both GHI and PHI are open to scrutiny.

Features Favorable to a Multi-payor Healthcare System in the United States

As mentioned above, the U.S. healthcare system already has many features in common with existing and successful multi-payor universal healthcare systems among OECD countries. GHI is functioning and knows its given role in the healthcare business. The government has already defined vulnerable populations: the very poor are covered by Medicaid, needy children are covered by SCHIPS, the elderly are covered by Medicare, and veterans and the military are covered by the Veterans Administration and other government coverage. There may be some debate as to the appropriateness of these decisions; but these decisions have been made, and these programs are more or less functional.

The U.S. has a vigorous PHI industry. There are several health insurance carriers and several methods for insurance carriers to be organized; indemnity insurance, HMOs, PPOs, mutual insurance companies, and corporate self-insurance plans. There is an active market for health insurance policies. Purchasers of PHI may purchase coverage individually or collectively through employment or through some other association. Given the regulatory parameters in which health insurers operate, they are flexible, numerous and competitive.

PHI covers a substantial proportion of the U.S. population. The U.S. Census Bureau estimates that approximately 70% of U.S. citizens with healthcare coverage have PHI (2003 estimate).[3] The result of a vigorous health insurance industry is that there is an active market for medical services with infrastructure capable of providing sophisticated state-of-the-art medical therapies without prolonged waiting times. Co-payments and deductibles have an effect on utilization and regulate moral hazard to a degree acceptable to the market and profitable to health insurers. These features of both GHI and PHI are favorable to a successful multi-payor system.

Features Unfavorable to a Multi-payor Healthcare System in the United States

There are, however, conditions both in the GHI sector and in the PHI sector of the health insurance market that are unfavorable to universal healthcare. In the GHI sector, there is, almost by definition, a disconnect between the revenue stream and the cost of services; GHI is funded based on tax revenues, thus forcing GHI to contain the amount of medical services it provides dependent upon its tax revenue-based budget. There is a further disconnect realized in the case of Medicaid, wherein the federal government retains authority but only partially funds benefits; a partially funded mandate is laid upon states to provide healthcare for the poor. And in the case of both Medicaid and Medicare, supply side control in the form of fee setting affects the willingness of providers to accept patients from these groups.

In the PHI sector the following unfavorable conditions affect the distribution of medical services, especially relative to conditions referred to by economists as "the essential conditions" for a commodity to be distributed in a competitive market. These are:

- *Lack of uniformity of product*
- *Lack of universal availability*
- *Lack of easy entry into the market*
- *Imperfect knowledge of product and price*
- *Lack of price sensitivity.*

These departures from the "essential conditions" manifest themselves in such practices as risk ratings, bundling of primary, complementary and supplementary insurance policies, and differential pricing, whether based on risk or on administrative costs. Market failure in regard to healthcare services hinges so critically upon the failed relationship between these practices and these essential conditions that these conditions will be the major element of discussion in the following chapter.

Without appropriate regulations to establish a level playing field, PHI cannot accomplish its defined policy goals. Among OECD member countries, regulations aimed specifically at implementing these "essential conditions" have met with varying degrees of success, often dependent upon how successful policy has been at supporting and protecting the essential elements. As has already been mentioned, in the absence of regulations prohibiting risk-based price discrimination, if one insurer applies risk rating methods, others must follow in order to remain competitive. But we have also seen that in OECD countries where risk rating methods are prohibited, insurers can and do compete successfully. Thus these kinds of regulations benefit the populations who most need medical services, and it is these kinds of regulations, evenly enforced, that level the playing field for PHI providers, allowing them to participate in achieving policy goals.

Conclusion

Regulations supportive of competitive market conditions are essential to a successful multi-payor universal healthcare system. They are the natural result of a goal-oriented definition of specific roles for both GHI and PHI, and are the reflection of policy based on goals relative to solvency and access.

It should go without saying that policy goals will necessarily require regulations favorable to competitive markets — regulations supportive of the essential elements of competitive markets so that a commodity like health insurance can be universally distributed in a competitive manner.

Selvoy M. Fillerup, MD, MSPH, FACS

CHAPTER SIX

Things Your Economist Assumes You Already Know

In a normally functioning market any willing buyer may buy the commodity for sale at a competitive price, and sellers increase revenues by selling increased quantities of the commodity. Take special note. In a <u>normal</u> market <u>any willing buyer</u> may buy the commodity that is for sale — all he or she needs is the cash to do so.

Market failure occurs when buyers cannot get the goods and services they need and want at competitive prices. In a failed market, sellers increase revenues not by increasing sales and market share, but by selecting the buyers to whom they will sell and by selling at high prices. Some buyers cannot get the commodity at any price! The United States health insurance market is just such a failed market.

One result of a failed market is the development of non-competitive high prices. Both the medical services markets and the health insurance markets in the United States demonstrate the signs of market failure.

As described previously, some of the nations of the OECD rely on competitive markets to provide health insurance to substantial proportions of their populations. In those nations, where the cost of healthcare is substantially lower than in the United States, healthcare markets are arguably more successful. How exactly are those markets different than the United States' health insurance market?

The following is a review of some basic features of markets generally and some peculiar features of medical services relative to market conditions.

Market Principles

Americans generally have confidence that competitive market economies are successful. This perception derives from the failure of almost all non-market economies, the most glaring example being the collapse of the former Soviet Union. *Ipso facto*, capitalism works; market economies are the first choice for any society wishing to promote prosperity among its citizens.

We are left to wonder then, if market economies generate such successes, why does the United States healthcare system have such an awkward relationship with competitive market methods? Why do we have so many different programs and so many regulations? And why can't the regulators just let us alone to enjoy market efficiencies in the business of medicine?

The typical response to these questions is a history lesson reviewing the piecemeal development of the long list of the various United States public and private healthcare programs, accompanied by a review of the economic and political circumstances that prompted each development. An alternate approach, taken here, is to review how a complex commodity — healthcare — responds, or rather fails to respond, to the requirements of a competitive market situation.

For any commodity to be distributed efficiently and equitably in a competitive market system, that commodity (or service) needs to meet certain conditions. Economists refer to these as the "essential conditions for perfect competition." These conditions define a "normal" market. In the absence of these conditions, an unregulated market will fail to provide efficient distribution of commodities and services. Economists refer to this as "market failure." The fact that medical services seldom meet these essential conditions is, in part, the reason for the wide variety of programs and regulations (HMOs, PPOs, tax incentives, private insurance, Medicare, Medicaid, the VA system, the State Children's Health Insurance Program, and so on) in the United States healthcare system today.

These essential conditions of a "normal" market are:
- *uniformity of product*
- *universal availability and/or transportability of goods and services*
- *easy entry to and exit from the market*
- *perfect knowledge of product and price*
- *price sensitivity.*

In addition to these traditionally discussed conditions there are two additional assumptions made about competitive markets of importance in the discussion of healthcare. These are:

- *the consumer is independent and pays the full price of goods and services, and*
- *anyone who wants to buy those goods or services may buy them without restriction.*

Arguably, it is because medical services are so poorly suited to free market conditions that institutions such as third party payors and governments, both state and federal, have resorted to price management, regulations, and even restrictions on who may purchase insurance. Certainly, the present system provides a high level of care for those with access, but healthcare access in the United States is not universal and it is increasingly expensive. Basic and even critical care is denied to many citizens. Americans, on average, live shorter lives than their European or Japanese counterparts, and the cost per capita for healthcare in the United States is nearly twice the cost in European systems. Year after year, we are spending more and getting less. Regulations mount, paperwork and frustrations increase. Yet any expectation that reliance solely on competitive market forces will remedy healthcare distribution is falsely founded.

Unregulated market systems are never expected to provide "universal" distribution of any commodity or service. With this in mind, those who desire universal healthcare ought never to expect that universal healthcare will be possible through a purely competitive market system. It is important to keep in mind, however, that a completely regulated healthcare system, in the absence of any market forces, presents its own set of problems.

I. A Review of the "Essential Conditions of Competitive Markets"

Unregulated markets, at least in economists' models, have certain distinguishing features that allow them to function. Understanding of these features, often referred to as the "essential characteristics" of competitive markets, is important to understanding the difficulties of distributing medical services in competitive markets. The remainder of this chapter is devoted to a discussion of these features.

A. Uniformity of Product

"Uniformity of product" refers to commodities that are uniform like beans, wheat, or any other relatively uniform product such as crude oil, or cotton, or steel. Tons of beans are available on the open market and are traded daily and always for the lowest price available. Any particular bean is pretty much like every other bean. Any ton of beans is pretty much like any other ton of beans. The product is uniform. It does not matter whether the beans were raised in North Dakota or Arkansas; beans are beans. This is uniformity of product, and this is one feature that makes the bean market a competitive market.

Doctors' visits, however, are not inherently uniform, nor are patients' needs. One patient may need a blood pressure check and a medication refill. The next patient may require x-rays, lab tests and a thorough physical exam. The resources and decisions required in each visit are different.

In spite of the many common aspects of medical training, physicians differ in their philosophies and practice methods. One doctor may be aggressive about counseling patients to exercise and lose weight; another may not feel the same urgency about weight loss. Specialty training generates different skill sets among physicians. Physicians are, after all, human, and should be expected to differ from one another. The time a patient spends in an office will vary from one doctor to the next; fees will differ from one doctor to another. Whether we like it or not, patients' needs and doctors' visits are not like beans; they are not uniform.

When a uniform commodity is sold in an open market, it is sold on the basis of price. Because every unit of the commodity is the same as every other unit, we can buy the lowest priced unit and get the same quality and the same convenience as with any other unit. But with healthcare services, there are considerations other than price. Purchasing decisions are based on convenience, location, and reputation; they are based on which insurance plans are accepted, or on the availability of an open appointment.

It is, therefore, no surprise that doctors' visits are not traded on a commodities market like so many tons of beans. Market forces do not affect the price or distribution of medical services the same way they affect uniform goods, and therefore market efficiencies are not realized for medical services as they are for other goods, like wheat, beans, clothing or paper.

B. Universal Availability and/or Transportability

The bean example demonstrates another feature about open markets — universal availability and/or transportability of product.

For example, a bean buyer in Dallas could get beans from almost anywhere, from California to Minnesota to Oklahoma. Beans are easily transported, and because they are so easily transported and do not change during transit, price dictates the location of origin.

Doctors' office visits, however, are not so easily transported. When a sack of beans is shipped, the same beans arrive: not so with doctors' visits. The information gathered from previous visits, the relationship, the confidence, and the first-hand understanding that are all part of a patient-doctor relationship cannot be transported to a new clinic and a new doctor along with the patient chart. Something is always left behind. New trust has to be built; new familiarity has to become part of a new relationship. All this takes time and, therefore, adds expense; lab tests and x-rays must be reviewed and new examinations performed.

Nor is medical expertise universally available. Specialists are not distributed uniformly around cities, or states, or around the country. The most sophisticated treatments are available only in medical centers in metropolitan areas. Highly trained specialists gather in and around the most technically advanced and forward thinking research centers. The expertise in one center differs from that of another center. One center may have the world's premier faculty in oncology, another may have expertise in genetics, a third may excel in organ transplants. There will likely always be differences in expertise from one center to another just as there are differences between metropolitan and rural medical facilities. Simply stated, there is no universal availability of medical services.

To the degree that physician visits are less available, less portable and less uniform than other products, they fail to meet the requirements of a competitive market. Just as the uniformity, and universal availability, and transportability of beans make their distribution in an open market very successful, and keep the price of beans low and competitive, the lack of these qualities in healthcare makes healthcare services unsuitable for distribution in a free market and makes their price unpredictable.

C. Easy Entry to and Exit from the Market Place

Very few commodities completely meet the next essential condition of an open market model, which is easy entry to and exit from the marketplace. Even bean farmers have barriers to entry into the marketplace. To successfully enter the bean market a farmer must have land, and a fairly large piece of land. And the farmer must have seed, tractors, and combines for harvest, and trucks to haul the beans to market. The farmer must know that there is a storage facility for his beans and trains that can carry the beans to buyers. These logistic hurdles are termed "barriers to market entry." To some degree, they limit the tonnage of beans available to the market at any one time.

There are many other kinds of barriers to market entry. Patents, licenses, permits, taxes, land use regulations, environmental laws, and certifications of competency are all barriers to market entry. Patents protect the first innovators of new products from competition; patents are therefore a barrier to market entry. Barbers must have licenses, liquor stores must have permits, many businesses must pay fees or special taxes or be bonded to stay in business, certain agricultural practices such as feedlots must be a certain distance from streams or communities, barbers must pass competency evaluations.

All manner of similar barriers exist in the medical industry. Not everyone who wants to sell pills or practice medicine is allowed to do so. Drug companies are required to demonstrate the effectiveness and safety of new products. Licenses are granted for medical devices, both to protect inventors and to assure that new devices are safe, reliable and effective. Regulations exist to monitor the safety and cleanliness of hospitals and to assure the performance and competence of staff. Enforcement of these regulations is accomplished by removal of licensure. If a hospital fails to maintain certain standards, the hospital can be closed.

Not just anyone is allowed to prescribe medications. The public expects that physicians and surgeons are educated in medicine, trained in their specialty fields, pass examinations certifying competence, and undergo licensing and monitoring for ethical and competent behavior. Medical and nursing schools must meet certain standards before they receive accreditation.

Hospital medical staffs screen applicants and limit their members to those they consider qualified.

We consider all these barriers to be protective, but they also regulate the numbers of producers of services; and they certainly limit the general availability of some services and products. Though not necessarily a protective barrier, even the cost of medical training is, for many, a barrier to entry into the medical professions.

Many services in the healthcare industry fail to meet the criteria of easy entry to the marketplace; these services cannot be expected to respond to typical market forces of supply and demand. As a consequence of regulating quality, supply is also regulated and price is affected.

D. Perfect Knowledge of Product and Price

Even when products or services are somewhat less uniform than beans, if there is sufficient knowledge about the quality and price of products, a buyer may be able to make informed buying decisions and get a good price for the value he receives. Almost everyone has an idea of what a really good lawn-mowing job looks like. If the first lawn service does a less than exemplary job on the lawn, the owner of the yard may seek the services of a second lawn care service, probably for a similar price. Automobiles, while different in some ways, are similar in many other ways, and a buyer may shop and compare, thus obtaining a relatively complete knowledge of features, quality and price.

But a visit to the Intensive Care Unit is not that way. Neither is a simple visit for a health check up.

No one knows, when going into an intensive care unit, what the procedures will be, what the tests will be, or what the final costs will be. There is no time to shop around. Even the doctor who places the patient into the ICU probably does not shop for an ICU based on price. The doctor will admit the patient to an ICU that is sufficiently convenient for both the doctor and the patient, one that can provide a nursing staff that is competent and reliable, a facility where the doctor has privileges and access to the services that the patient requires. The patient seldom has any knowledge of the costs of these services. In short, there is limited knowledge of both product and price on the part of the patient when entering an ICU, or for that matter, when entering an emergency room or a surgical suite or any physician's office.

One may rely upon regulations to assure the quality of these services, or one may make assumptions about the qualifications and good intentions of the nursing staff, the lab, the x-ray team, and so on. But with respect to price, from hospital to hospital, and from one insurance carrier to another, and from one clinic to another, accounting models vary and prices vary. It is very difficult for any patient to discover the reasons for the differences in prices among the same medical services. This holds for almost any medical service that one could name.

That there is some competition between hospitals based on price might be argued, but others would argue that under current conditions of price negotiation and regulation, hospitals struggle to meet expenses and therefore attempt to raise prices at every opportunity. In either case, when dealing with medical services, the ability of the consumer to shop and compare services based on quality and price is limited; the subsequent lack of perfect knowledge about product and price eliminates nearly all medical services from any likelihood that they could be traded openly.

E. Price Sensitivity

The concept of price sensitivity is simple. Price sensitivity exists if, when the price of a product is lowered, sales go up or, when the price goes up, sales go down. If the price of gasoline is low, one might take a trip. If chicken is cheap, one might buy some extra and put it in the freezer. Conversely, if the price of cars goes up, the old car gets driven a few extra miles.

This, however, is seldom the situation with medical services. If a person does not have high blood pressure, that person will not need or want to buy medicine for blood pressure — no matter how low the price goes. And if a person does have high blood pressure and the price of blood pressure medications drop, that person is still not likely to buy more blood pressure medication than is required. Furthermore, even when the price of blood pressure medicine goes up, that person still needs to buy the same required amount. The amount of blood pressure medicine a person purchases is not sensitive to price.

With many medical conditions, urgency is of greater significance than price. A person needing an appendectomy needs it right now, regardless of cost.

Confronted with such a situation, the relative value of the appendectomy is very high; it is literally worth a life — the likelihood of death from untreated appendicitis is far too real. And a person never needs more than one appendectomy, so even if the price comes down, no one buys two. Furthermore, a person would not normally go shopping for, or buy, an appendectomy even if the price were very cheap. It will only be purchased when absolutely needed. Once again, the buying patterns and buying reasons for individual medical services are seldom price sensitive. Conceivably, the price of any emergency service could be extremely high.

Prices in the medical field are not set exclusively by market conditions associated with supply and demand. In the business of medicine, prices are artificially set; in some situations prices are based on the cost of overhead plus a certain percentage of mark-up. In many cases, third-party payors negotiate with providers for even lower prices for medical services.

Because demand for medical services is not price sensitive, and because every method of setting prices is somewhat artificially derived, open market conditions cannot be expected to bring the prices of medical services into true supply and demand equilibrium.

II. Additional Assumptions Regarding Competitive Markets

The existence of insurance companies confounds two additional assumptions about competitive markets. The first assumption is that the consumer is independent and is responsible for payment of the full price of goods and services received; the second is that anyone who wants to buy those goods or services may buy them without restriction and at the same price offered to any other buyer.

First of all, health insurance introduces the insurance company as an intermediate between buyers and sellers of medical services — as a third party payor — and, in essence, hides the price of medical services from patients. In this arrangement the patient, or the buyer, is not independent and seldom pays the full price of medical services, but rather pays out-of-pocket only a fraction of the immediate cost of medical services. The perception is that the insurance company pays the balance.

Because patients pay only a fraction of immediate costs, they are inclined to use more medical services than they might use if they paid the full price of services at the time they were rendered — to over-utilize. This effect, historically referred to as "moral hazard," is measurable, and it affects the cost of insurance without necessarily improving community health. Insurance companies have responded to over-utilization with the relatively successful strategy of imposing co-payments and deductibles so that patients must pay a large enough portion of their immediate costs that they do not use medical services without some sensitivity to price. (But remember that while co-payments and deductibles have been shown to decrease utilization rates, they may also discourage patients from appropriate utilization.)

Arguably, however, many consumers of health insurance no longer consider the prices of individual medical services but instead consider their costs for a health benefits package — the cost of health insurance plus out-of-pocket expenses. This "package" becomes the commodity. Certainly, individuals do not go out for the afternoon shopping for an appendectomy or a cardiac bypass based on price. (That function has been assumed by the insurance industry.) Rather, they shop for health insurance policies, generally negotiated through employers.

Likewise, the providers of healthcare (hospitals, clinics and physicians) negotiate price with third party payors. The commodity of interest to both patients and providers is the *assurance* that medical services will be paid for, so that both patients and providers negotiate with health insurance companies based on price.

Secondly, with regard to the insurance industry, we no longer assume "guaranteed issue," which means that any willing buyer may buy the commodity at the offered price. Some individuals can be, and often are, refused health insurance. This is ultimately the result of insurers competing for clients with the lowest health risks. Insurers prefer to enroll healthy clients rather than unhealthy clients for obvious reasons and may simply refuse to sell a policy to patients with increased health risks. But if issue is guaranteed, any willing buyer may purchase insurance.

Years ago, insurers engaged in a practice referred to as community rating, which meant that they charged the same price for everyone of a given age and gender regardless of health status or group size. But administrative costs were greater for smaller groups and for individuals, and it soon became apparent that individuals seldom bought health insurance unless they thought they would use it, thus making individual purchasers more expensive to insure than members of large groups. Eventually insurers abandoned the practice of community rating, and individuals, small groups, and those with known illnesses were charged higher premiums. (It is arguable that with advances in electronic methods of record keeping that there is now very little difference in the cost of insuring a small vs. a large group, but the practice of charging lower prices for larger groups persists.)

The result has been the development of a wide variety of health insurance policies and prices as well as the placement of restrictions and conditions on purchasers of health insurance that favored healthier populations. Consumers no longer have the ability to purchase health insurance at a common price; individual consumers, especially those people who most need healthcare coverage, find themselves obligated to pay higher prices.

There are far reaching effects, both economically and socially, as a result of the fact that health insurance distorts these two assumptions about competitive markets: that the consumer is independent and is responsible for the full price of commodities, and that any consumer may buy the offered commodity for the market price.

Even though insurance companies, as third-party payors, distort the prices of individual medical services

— and therefore distort the consumption of those services — and even though all consumers are not presently offered the same prices for the same policies, it is worth remembering that insurance policies themselves, with their associated co-payments and deductibles, are now commonplace and are widely perceived to be a commodity.

Combining a policy of community rating with a policy assuring uniform minimum benefits, so that every insurance carrier offered the same uniform policy — or at least one basic uniform policy — at a competitive price in a competitive market, would introduce both uniformity of product regarding the commodity of health insurance and improve knowledge of price and product regarding healthcare services generally. Furthermore, if issue was guaranteed and enrollment was mandatory, the problem of portability would largely care for itself.

III. Review: Medical Services Do Not Meet the Essential Conditions Necessary for Distribution in a Competitive Market, but Health Insurance Could

The essential conditions of competitive marketplaces have been described. It is important to remember that the standard market models that are so effective in bringing fresh fruit to our tables, reliable automobiles into our garages, and a wide variety of colorful clothing to our closets are well suited to commodities that can be traded in competitive markets. The price of any given brand of shirts is similar in Denver and Chicago. The price and quality of eggs in Dallas is similar to the price and quality of eggs in Pittsburgh. Although the essential characteristics are, in reality, seldom all present together for any given commodity, enough of them are present in enough commodities that our market economy continues to flourish.

But medical goods and services are quirky; they do not match any of the conditions for a competitive market.

The seed of frustration with the current situation in the business of medicine lies not only in the details of the patched–together network that has evolved in America, but also in our inconsistent thinking about competitive markets. The commodities of beans and medical services are worlds apart.

But the health insurance market is not so very far from markets for commodities such as beans. Health insurance can be marketed much more like a commodity than can individual medical services, as will be shown in the following chapter. It becomes important, therefore, to distinguish between the markets for individual medical services and the market for health insurance.

> It becomes important, therefore, to distinguish between the markets for individual medical services and the market for health insurance.

True, the health insurance market is entirely dependent upon the cost of medical services because health insurance provides access to and pays for medical services; so the two markets, although they have fundamental differences, often appear to be the same market. Do not be misled. Health insurance and medical care are different services and different markets; the medical services purchased with dollars that pass through health insurance companies are subject to different market forces than are medical services purchased by individuals. Health insurers pay for large amounts of medical services based on actuarial predictions of need; an individual does not.

Restoring "normalcy" to the health insurance market opens the opportunity to have a multi-payor universal healthcare system with complementary roles for both PHI and GHI. Mending that market requires only that simple policies are implemented together: mandatory enrollment, community rating, guaranteed issue, and uniform benefits.

These policy concepts are critical to the observed success of other nations' healthcare systems. They have been discussed before and will be discussed again in future chapters.

Selvoy M. Fillerup, MD, MSPH, FACS

CHAPTER SEVEN

The Experiment

The United States is in an unusual position. The country appears to be at the close of a decades-long experiment testing whether a country without a national healthcare policy will be successful relative to a wide variety of systems that do have national healthcare policies. The result of this experiment is that the United States spends a higher percent of its GDP on healthcare than any other industrialized nation — a result that has financially hobbled American industries.

> The result of this experiment is that the United States spends a higher percent of its GDP on healthcare than any other industrialized nation — a result that has financially hobbled American industries.

With the expansion of the private health insurance industry during the 1940s and 1950s, the assurance that medical services would be paid for became a commodity. The value of this assurance became particularly apparent during the 1960s following the passage of Medicare and Medicaid legislation.

Combined, the elderly and the indigent populations constituted a large market. Huge sums of money flowed into medical services. With this new cash flow, the quantity and sophistication of medical services increased. Providers soon became attracted to the idea that they would be paid for the services they provided. Patients were attracted to the notion that medical expenses need not be financially devastating. Anyone who could sell that assurance had something to offer to both providers and patients. The private health insurance industry grew. Healthcare was a transformed industry.

Indeed, by the 1970s, anyone without health insurance faced a certain degree of financial risk, and those without health insurance began to affect providers' bottom lines.

The passage of Medicare and Medicaid in the 1960s was not unopposed. The political climate at that time in the United States was very much against socialized medicine — and against communism or socialism in almost any form. (America was actively fighting a communist regime in Vietnam.) President Lyndon Johnson had attempted to pass universal healthcare but had been opposed by almost every conservative political group in the nation, including the American Medical Association. Many Americans sneered at the British and Canadian "socialized" healthcare systems. That there were vocal proponents of universal healthcare is true, but they succeeded in obtaining tax-funded government healthcare only for the poor and the elderly. Universal enrollment in healthcare was not accomplished. Thus a private health insurance industry based upon a risk-mitigation philosophy became entrenched.

Divergent Paths for Private Health Insurance

At this time, there were already health insurance industries in many European nations. Interestingly, private health insurance in the United States took a different form than it did in Europe. In Europe, healthcare was considered a social or community responsibility. All healthcare coverage in Europe, private health insurance as well as government sponsored "socialized" programs, was structured so that it performed the role of cost redistribution. Healthcare coverage in the United States, however, took on the role of risk mitigation. In the United States, health insurance was the responsibility of the individual and only became an employment benefit when tax incentives were granted to employers who provided health insurance.

In Europe, health insurance was perceived as a social service and regulated accordingly. If enrollment in a national healthcare plan was not automatic, enrollment in some form of insurance was mandatory in every country. Community rating meant that persons with medical conditions could not be discriminated against by charging them higher premiums. Insurers could not deny coverage to anyone.

In the United States the health insurance product evolved differently. Insurance products in general are designed to reduce the risks associated with any venture in which the outcome is uncertain. The notion of ill health as an uncertain event against which a person could buy insurance became the premise under which health insurance was sold — health insurance was a risk-related product.

It quickly became apparent to insurers that it costs more money to insure a person with known health risks than a person without health risks. Consequently insurers discontinued the practice of community rating. Insurers could, and do, deny coverage to persons with a high likelihood of utilizing costly medical services.

The point of this discussion is not to point the finger of blame at the United States health insurance industry. Without a national policy to direct the underwriting policies of insurers, insurers in the United States are left with an environment in which they must compete on the basis of risk mitigation.

Three Healthcare Coverage Models

The point here is to clarify that private health insurance in the United States is a decidedly different product than it is in Europe and other member nations of the Organization for Economic Cooperation and Development (OECD). Following this distinction there are three categories into which healthcare coverage models may fall;

• *Government health insurance that accepts any enrollee regardless of health status (found in several countries in Europe and in the Medicare system in the United States),*

• *Private health insurance that accepts any enrollee regardless of health status (as is found in Europe), and*

- *Private health insurance that discriminates among enrollees based on the nature of health status (as is found in the United States).*

In the first two of these models, health insurance performs a cost redistribution function. In the third model, "the United States model," health insurance performs a risk-mitigation function.

There is nothing particularly immoral about insurance performing a risk-mitigation function; this merely represents the absence of national policy directing insurers to perform in any other way. The risk-mitigation model seems to be working just fine for home insurance, life insurance, auto insurance, and other forms of insurance. But in the realm of health insurance, the risk-mitigation model in the United States has proven itself to be very expensive.

In the United States both models exist. As noted above, Medicare functions as a cost redistribution model, and private health insurance functions as a risk-mitigation model. Notably, per capita administrative costs for Medicare are considerably less than administrative costs in the private health insurance industry even though Medicare spends more money on healthcare per enrollee than private insurance. Additionally, administrative costs among the nations of the OECD where private health insurance performs a cost redistribution function are lower than in the United States. Per capita health administration costs in 1999 in the United States were $1,059, more than triple the health administration cost of $307 per capita in Canada.[42]

For the past half-century, the three models have been running side by side in a global social experiment. The results are in:

- *Government healthcare programs that perform a cost redistribution function are able to contain administrative cost;*

- *Private health insurance, when regulated as a social service, performs a cost redistribution function and contains administrative cost; but*

- *Private health insurance, when left to operate as a risk-mitigation service, has substantially higher administrative costs.*

One might wonder what it is about the risk-mitigation model that increases per capita healthcare costs. The following topics should provide fodder for debate, but the reality of substantially higher healthcare care costs in the United States is not debatable.

The Hidden Costs of Avoiding Risk

Subtle factors affect administrative cost in the risk-mitigation model. The first is the need for health insurers under this model to identify and avoid risk. It is acknowledged that insurers using this model spend substantial amounts of money deciding who will be covered and at what price. The actuarial industry, which performs the function of assessing risk and its cost, is expensive. Profits in this model come from avoiding unnecessary risk or from charging high premiums for accepting high risks. The entire process of assessing and avoiding risk adds to administrative costs in this model.

Artificial Elevation of Medical Costs

A second factor affecting cost in the risk-mitigation model is the cost of medical services. Ironically, insurers in this model increase profits when the costs of covered medical services are high — at least high enough that insurees desire and purchase health insurance to mitigate the risk of encountering those costs.

Health insurance becomes more valuable as the financial risk associated with high medical costs increases. Thus the value of health insurance increases as medical costs rise. Consequently, health insurers can charge high premiums and stand to earn greater profits as the cost of medical care rises.

The insurance industry has made few efforts to limit the amount of medical services used or the costs of medical care. Why not? Contemplate "game theory." At first glance, it would seem that when insurers paid lower amounts for medical services they would stand to earn greater profits. But if medical costs are low, individuals need not be concerned about the financial risk associated with medical care. Only when medical care is expensive is health insurance valuable. It is therefore to the advantage of insurers to continue to pay for expensive medical services; high prices for medical services increase the demand for health insurance. And as long as insurers are willing, at least to some degree, to sustain high prices for medical services, provider will expect to receive high fees. Whether this effect is the result of intentional collusion or merely the effect of the wrong incentive misdirecting an "invisible hand," the result is the same.

Uncertainty

Uncertainty about the financial risk associated with medical care is the engine for profits in the insurance industry and consequently for high fees for medical services.

It is arguable that this cycle is broken under conditions of universal enrollment. Universal healthcare reduces uncertainty. In every country with universal enrollment, the cost of medical services and of health insurance is substantially lower than in the United States; the per capita healthcare costs in OECD countries are on average 40.9% the per capita healthcare cost of the United States.[43]

People in countries with universal healthcare live under an umbrella of assurance: medical care will be provided at reasonable prices and health insurance premiums reflect this generalized confidence. Citizens have no apprehensions about potentially devastating high medical costs. The relative value of private health insurance is diminished, and therefore its price falls. Insurers have no incentive to sustain providers in their expectations of receiving high fees. The case in point for this argument is Switzerland, where there is no government healthcare program; enrollment in private health insurance is mandatory and per capita healthcare costs are about 30% less than they are in the United States.

Side by Side in the USA

In the United States, a cost redistribution model and a risk mitigation model operate side by side with conflicting incentives: Medicare (which seeks to avoid high costs for medical services, having no profit incentive) and the United States private health insurance industry (which, for the reasons described above, tolerates relatively high costs for medical services). The reaction of the healthcare market is interesting.

Forty five percent of the total of money flowing through the healthcare system comes through public funds; about one third of this, or 16% of the total, comes through Medicare. Providers cannot ignore such a large market.

But the privately insured patient, through the insurance carrier, pays for services at a higher rate than the Medicare patient. These higher payments induce providers and hospitals to preferentially serve private paying patients, and generate expectations of higher fees for medical services. In response, Medicare sets fixed fees for services in order to avoid a bidding competition for medical services and offers those fees on take-it-or-leave-it basis. If Medicare were not such a large segment of the market, it would likely be compelled to either raise its fees (which it actually does, at least to some degree, and not because of market demands but because of political pressure!) or impose additional regulations in order to find providers willing to accept these lower fees. As it is, providers who can avoid accepting new Medicare patients actually do so.

The point here is that when a risk-mitigation model (U.S. style private health insurance) operates concurrently with a cost-redistribution model (Medicare), there are market pressures through the former for higher prices for medical services that must be dealt with by the latter.

Compare the United States' situation to that of nations such as the Netherlands or Japan where both government healthcare programs and private health insurance are structured to accomplish cost distribution functions regarding healthcare services. In 2000, the per capita healthcare cost in the Netherlands was approximately US$2,250 compared to the United States' cost of $4,500. In Japan, per capita costs were barely over US$2,000 for the same year.[43]

Conclusion

Uncertainty is expensive; the greater the uncertainty, the greater the expense of mitigating uncertainty.

Universal enrollment diminishes uncertainty for insurers (as well as providers and patients), thereby reducing administrative and actuarial costs, and may indirectly reduce costs for medical services. Indeed, where healthcare has been considered a public service to be administered under a cost redistribution model, whether that administration is by government or by private industry, the costs of administration and even the costs of medical services have been lower than under a risk-mitigation model.

In many ways the United States is in an enviable position. It has a strong and competent private health insurance industry. It has a vigorous healthcare infrastructure with excellent hospitals and training facilities and absolutely remarkable technology. But its risk-mitigation model for health insurance has failed. This model arguably contributes to increased medical costs and definitely contributes to increased administrative costs for health insurance.

The redefinition of the role of private health insurance in the United States can be accomplished by enacting a national healthcare policy focused on a cost redistribution model. The cost redistribution model, whether it is called socialized medicine, or social justice, or simply universal healthcare, has demonstrated the capacity to significantly reduce per capita healthcare costs.

> The cost redistribution model, whether it is called socialized medicine, or social justice, or simply universal healthcare, has demonstrated the capacity to significantly reduce per capita healthcare costs.

Americans must, of course, decide whether to change to a single-payor healthcare system or retain their private health insurance industry. But if the private health insurance industry is preserved it must be provided an environment wherein it can perform cost redistribution functions rather than risk-mitigation functions.

As stated previously, the policy measures that will accomplish this goal are universal enrollment, a uniform minimum healthcare benefits package offered by all insurers, guaranteed issue, and community ratings.

Selvoy M. Fillerup, MD, MSPH, FACS

CHAPTER EIGHT

This Looks Do-able

Universal enrollment in a healthcare system is at once a moral and an economic objective. The policy instruments of community rating, guaranteed issue, and uniform benefits go only so far in achieving the economic benefits of universal healthcare. Interestingly, perhaps amazingly, these policies, in the absence of a policy for universal enrollment, cannot lower health insurance or healthcare costs. We have seen two methods of achieving universal enrollment: default universal enrollment and mandatory universal enrollment. Either way, the means and advantages of achieving universal enrollment are tightly knit into the fabric of normal market economics.

No industrial country in the world has a completely competitive market system for healthcare delivery, not Switzerland, not the Netherlands, not Germany, not Japan, and certainly not the United States, where the so-called healthcare system is a patchwork of related healthcare programs and regulations. Some level of subsidy and regulation has evolved in every system.

Even so, there are advantages to competitive market systems that should not be ignored. Competitive markets foster innovation in science and technology, in management methods and in competitive pricing. And because these advantages have improved the availability of so many commodities and services, Americans are justifiably slow to abandon these advantages for a socialized single-payor system.

Likewise, there are certain disadvantages to government-managed systems that have been demonstrated among other nations that the United States would do well to avoid. As has been shown, universal healthcare does not necessarily mean government healthcare. If a sustainable, universal healthcare system is to evolve in the United States, the challenge will be to generate regulations that foster market efficiencies applicable to healthcare services while simultaneously promoting universal healthcare coverage.

Universal Healthcare: Not Necessarily Single-payor Healthcare

Universal healthcare is certainly feasible (twenty-nine of the world's thirty industrialized countries have found ways to accomplish this), and universal healthcare would be an economic benefit to the citizens of the United States in many ways. All that is required is objectivity regarding the advantages of the basic principles of market economics and the implementation of basic regulations to enhance market efficiencies where healthcare services are concerned.

We have shown that medical services are not easily distributed using a competitive market system; they do not meet the necessary criteria for distribution in a competitive market. Of particular interest are three practices related to the insurance industry that deserve description. These are uniformity of product, community rating, and guaranteed issue.

Uniformity of Product: As discussed in Chapter Six, medical services in particular do not naturally constitute a "uniform product." Immunizations are different from x-ray studies which are different from doctors' office visits which are different from surgeries.

Interestingly, much of profitability in any market derives from the antithesis of uniformity — namely "product differentiation." In the case of health insurance, however, product differentiation is not beneficial to consumers or providers, nor is it beneficial to society generally. It is, nevertheless, a feature of the health insurance market in the United States.

Healthcare insurance policies differ in the breadth of coverage they offer, the waiting times required for pre-existing conditions, co-payments required, and limits on coverage; and, inevitably, there is a different panel of doctors, nurses, and other providers associated with each HMO, PPO, or other provider panel.

But if all insurance companies were to offer at least one policy that was uniform — a standard minimum basic benefits package (MBBP) regarding covered services — we would then have <u>uniformity of product</u>

regarding health insurance policies. Then the health insurance market place would begin to enjoy the advantages that naturally follow when uniform products, such as wheat or beans, are sold in their competitive markets.

Then, because buyers would have improved knowledge of the product they were buying (buyers would know they were receiving identical healthcare benefits regardless of the company from whom the policy was purchased) they could shop for healthcare benefits based on price, and insurance companies would compete based on price in order to sell policies.

Community Rating: Years ago, insurers engaged in the practice referred to as community rating, which meant that they charged the same price for everyone regardless of age, gender or health status. But administrative costs were greater for smaller groups, and for individuals, and it soon became apparent that individuals seldom bought health insurance unless they thought they would use it, thus making individual purchasers riskier and more expensive to insure.

Eventually insurers abandoned the practice of community rating; administrative costs were lower for large groups, and individuals were largely priced out of the market or refused coverage because they were a higher insurance risk generally. One result was the development of a wide variety of health insurance policies and prices. Implementing the practice of community rating as a matter of national healthcare policy would now be required in order to establish a standard healthcare coverage package available to all citizens without price differentiation. Indeed, insurers could only implement community ratings if community ratings were enforced as part of a national healthcare policy creating a level playing field for all insurers.

Guaranteed Issue: The term "guaranteed issue" is not new in the insurance industry. We have seen in many OECD countries that guaranteed issue specifically prohibits insurers from denying coverage based on health status.

When combined, community ratings and guaranteed issue assure that healthcare costs are distributed across the entire population and not refused to those who most need healthcare services.

Advantages of Uniformity of Product, Community Ratings, and Guaranteed Issue

Price sensitivity: The practices of uniformity of product, community ratings and guaranteed issue are not new ideas; they are simple practices that have been incorporated into the regulatory framework of several OECD countries and could easily become part of healthcare policy in the United States. One purpose of implementing these policies is to bring price sensitivity to the healthcare market. When prices become sensitive to demand, they usually become lower.

As discussed previously, uniformity of product and universal availability are market conditions that support competitive pricing, and in the case of health insurance, lower prices — or at least competitive prices — for health insurance will make health insurance more affordable for those who most need healthcare. The benefits of price sensitivity and how it is achievable in the health insurance market will be discussed further in Chapter Nine. Simply keep in mind that uniformity of product, community ratings, and guaranteed issue are important policy tools that can make this possible.

The healthcare industry is in an excellent position to market uniform health insurance policies; already the insurance industry develops and sells uniform health insurance policies to large groups and corporations. The idea only needs to be expanded upon so that a standard policy is sold by all insurers. What is lacking is a standard upon which all insurers can, or must, agree — the minimum basic benefits package (MBBP).

The task of defining a standard MBBP is, in the context of a universal healthcare policy, suitable to the role of government; the establishment of a standard health insurance policy will only be accomplished if that goal is accepted as a national responsibility and incorporated into a national healthcare policy. The OECD experience has shown — notably in the Netherlands and in Switzerland, but in other countries as well — that when a uniform MBBP is offered, insurers do compete based on price. When this happens, health insurance becomes price sensitive, and health insurance costs reach market equilibrium.[4]

Once an MBBP is defined, it would thereafter be the opportunity of health insurance companies to provide an array of "complementary" or "supplementary" policies with expanded coverage for additional services. However, an MBBP offered by all health insurers will introduce favorable market forces and market efficiencies, including price sensitivity and price competition, to the healthcare industry.

Universal Availability: Another concept important to competitive markets is referred to variably as "portability," or "transportability," or "universal availability" of product. Portability has been a sticky issue for insurees because of the complexities of assuring that healthcare benefits will be available when changing careers. But if an MBBP is uniform and community rated, and if issue is guaranteed, workers could change employers and careers without concern about having healthcare benefits. A worker could leave a career in California and accept a new position in Virginia and know that he could obtain the same health benefits at a competitive price.

Regarding portability, there are several theoretical advantages to both individuals and societies when healthcare benefits are universally available. Two of these are related to mobility of the workforce. First, with universal availability of healthcare benefits, workers are free to seek rewarding employment wherever they choose without fear of losing benefits. Second, employers can compete for productive workers without concerns about the ability to match health insurance benefits. The ensuing advantage to society generally is that a talented workforce becomes more productive when employers are free to match job opportunities to employees' skills, thereby increasing the adaptability and productivity of the workforce. These and other benefits will be discussed further in Chapter Eleven.

The only regulations needed to gain the advantages of these two market conditions are:

- *that a uniform MBBP be defined*
- *that it be available under conditions of community ratings*
- *that issue is guaranteed*
- *that universal enrollment is mandatory.*

Insurance companies already have sophisticated information and information systems in place; it should be merely a matter of processing that information to determine the price at which they can offer the MBBP.

Providing Default Enrollment

It is a misconception that all the uninsured in the United States are too poor to afford insurance or too ill to be satisfactory insurance risks. Even though many of the uninsured cite cost as the reason they remain uninsured, most are employed; and in most cases employers and employees could share the cost of health insurance. About 88% of the uninsured live in households where one or more persons are employed, and most live in homes with adequate incomes: 53% of the uninsured have incomes greater than $40,000 per year and 75% have incomes greater than $20,000 per year. Most are healthy: 92% report their health status to be either "excellent," "good," or "very good."[7] The present uninsured population is largely "insurable."

Vulnerable populations — the elderly and the very poor — are already covered by government programs.

But another group — a "quasi-vulnerable" group, the working poor — requires additional attention. Under a multi-payor system, this fraction of the population still requires government involvement in healthcare coverage. This includes uninsured and under-insured workers, who, in the United States, are often part-time employees, the self-employed, and temporary employees.

It is apparent that the three conditions of uniformity of product, community ratings, and guaranteed issue are not sufficient by themselves to guarantee universal healthcare. A fourth condition is needed — automatic, or default, enrollment.

> The three conditions of Uniformity of product, Community ratings, and Guaranteed issue are not sufficient by themselves to guarantee universal healthcare. A fourth condition is needed -- automatic, or default, enrollment.

Medicare insures the elderly, Medicaid insures the very poor, and the VA insures eligible veterans, but there is no specified enrollment plan for those who are self-employed, or who are temporary employees, or who work in industries that simply do not provide healthcare benefits. Many are left to struggle with higher premiums or higher co-payments or other forms of price discrimination for their healthcare coverage.

This group is addressed in Japan in much the same way the Japanese have addressed those employed in their agricultural sector; they are simply insured through a partnership with the government. Japanese agriculture workers, self employed workers and those employed in small businesses contribute to their own insurance and pay a fixed proportion of their insurance costs.[4,33,34]

In France, the working poor are provided the same benefits as the rest of the population, for which they pay through consumption taxes, but they are also provided complementary insurance as a separate consideration.

In Switzerland, all citizens purchase health insurance by mandate, but individuals are allowed to apply to the government to assist with payment of premiums when they cannot pay.

In each of these instances, the issue of poverty is considered as an issue separate from the issue of universal health coverage — basic healthcare coverage is mandatory, poverty is addressed as its own issue.

In Canada, Great Britain, Scandinavia, Germany, and the Netherlands and in other countries with universal GHI, default enrollment is not an issue; it is the norm.

The real issue under consideration in the United States is that a fraction of the population is simply unable or unwilling to enroll for PHI, either for financial or personal reasons. In order to attain universal coverage, and in the absence of other compulsory means, government remains the only entity capable of providing default enrollment for this group.

Premiums for Default Enrollment

If the economic and social benefits of universal coverage are to be realized, there must be a planned mechanism of enrollment for the working poor — and for any others who prefer to enroll in GHI. Only through some form of default enrollment policy can universal healthcare enrollment be achieved.

The issue of default or mandatory enrollment in an insurance plan has been debated before. The alternatives to default enrollment in a multi-payor system include continuation of cost-shifting; or tax subsidized medical care for everyone not enrolled in PHI. Continued cost-shifting means that providers must leave in place all the offices and operations currently employed to perform the tasks of cost-shifting. This would achieve nothing; it is essentially the status quo. And if a tax subsidized coverage is available and there is no cost to enroll by default, default enrollment would immediately appear to be free health insurance. Default enrollment for free healthcare would suddenly be the preferred means of obtaining coverage! A multi-payor system would become a tax-subsidized single-payor GHI system as quickly as people could abandon PHI!

At issue then, if a multi-payor plan is to be proposed, is how to provide default enrollment but still prevent healthcare from becoming a tax subsidized entitlement for everyone. In order to do this, even unwilling enrollees must assist in the payment of their own healthcare premiums. It is important at this point to consider that one of the primary purposes of assigning a policy role to PHI is to relieve government of the

> At issue then, if a multi-payor plan is to be proposed, is how to provide default enrollment but still prevent healthcare from becoming a tax-subsidized entitlement for everyone.

responsibility of administering healthcare benefits to non-vulnerable populations. It is therefore important that it should be at least somewhat uncomfortable for non-vulnerable populations to accept default coverage through GHI.

A default enrollment program would mean the establishment of another organization under the auspices of GHI (in addition to, or perhaps in place of, Medicare, Medicaid and other already established programs). This program would look and act very much like an insurance company. This program would enroll non-vulnerable populations in a health insurance plan and would have authority to collect premiums from all enrollees.

There are at least two approaches to financing this program, at least in regard to the working poor. One approach would separate the issues of poverty and healthcare. Treat poverty under its own agenda; deal with poverty through tax relief or other benefits, but treat universal healthcare separately. Focus on the fact that a universal healthcare plan is intended to provide healthcare — not to correct the causes of poverty. Or to alleviate the effects of poverty. Or to correct other social inequities. Under this approach, every enrollee, including those who elected GHI for other reasons, would be required to participate in the cost of their healthcare coverage and would be charged the competitive price for their healthcare coverage. The working poor, or their insurance carriers, could apply for relief after the cost of their healthcare had been paid. (Those who are familiar with Earned Income Tax Credits will understand that the mechanisms to address this are already in place in the U.S.)[40]

In another approach, the newly formed GHI program would have authority to implement a sliding scale applicable to premium prices in order to accommodate citizens who did not qualify for Medicaid but whose income prohibited their paying full price for health insurance premiums. In short, this would be a government managed health insurance program with authority to means-test and charge accordingly. Submission to a means test would be the option available for all those who elected to enroll in GHI hoping to obtain reduced premiums.

These two alternatives merely constitute a choice regarding the timing of when a healthcare subsidy for the working poor is allowed. In the first approach it is allowed after the premium is paid; in the second approach the subsidy is calculated and awarded before the premium is paid.

Notably, when the subsidy is provided after the premium is paid, health policy makers may advance healthcare decisions independent of considerations of wealth or the lack thereof. This approach also places the responsibility for issues concerning unemployment, welfare and poverty into a different forum — a forum separate from healthcare.

The most readily available mechanism to accomplish either of these options is for government to collect a premium from GHI enrollees along with taxes. Income tax is mandatory; workers compensation insurance is mandatory; a default premium for GHI might also be mandatory. Accommodations for those whose incomes are low could be made through other forms of tax relief, but the price of the insurance premium should not be invisible even though it might not be completely felt. In this manner, non-vulnerable populations — those with adequate means to contribute to their own health premiums would find it to their advantage to enroll in PHI. Indeed, if a multi-payor universal healthcare system is to succeed, it ought to be at least as comfortable for non-vulnerable populations to enroll in PHI as in GHI.

Conclusion

The goal is universal healthcare. A multi-payor system appears practical, and there are economic and social advantages that make a multi-payor system attractive. If all U.S. citizens were enrolled in an insurance plan, most could be insured privately, either through work or individually. Those who were unable or unwilling to purchase insurance policies from private insurers would be enrolled for coverage under a government program offering the standard MBBP. Non-vulnerable populations could enroll for GHI, either by choice or by inaction, but would pay the premium for (be taxed for) their coverage. Those found to lack the capacity to pay for government coverage (under-employed or unemployed) could be subsidized through other tax-related allowances.

Because most of the uninsured have employment, there would be only a fraction of the entire non-elderly and non-Medicaid populations unable to contribute in some way to their health insurance costs. Thus, there would not be a significantly larger burden upon the government, or upon taxpayers, if the government defined the standard healthcare benefits package and then required that all employers share the cost to insure temporary and part-time employees through either a private or the government healthcare policy.

Universal enrollment is certainly achievable; others nations have done it already. But it is only achievable with a clearly stated healthcare policy, with clearly stated goals, and with regulations supportive of those goals.

Selvoy M. Fillerup, MD, MSPH, FACS

CHAPTER NINE

Show Me the Revenue Curve

Several models for providing universal healthcare have been shown in the preceding review of OECD countries' healthcare systems. These models illustrate how certain principles of policy determine increased success for achieving access and solvency. Specifically, PHI and GHI working in complementary roles achieve a favorable degree of success, especially when national policy directs PHI to accomplish public goals. This occurs partly because favorable changes in market dynamics accompany universal enrollment.

The United States, as discussed, does not yet have a policy for achieving universal healthcare enrollment. But suppose universal healthcare — within a framework of guaranteed issue and community ratings — was actually enacted in the U.S.; what would happen? Could the U.S. anticipate similar beneficial changes in market dynamics?

Keep in mind that everything is a tradeoff. Even sustaining the status quo exacts a cost, and that cost may be greater than one might imagine. We may see that the benefits of universal healthcare are well worth the change!

The Current Position of the United States

The United States already has in place many of the features of a successful multi-payer healthcare system: most of the population is privately insured, there are large numbers of competitive insurers, and there is variety among insurance carriers (PPOs, HMOs, indemnity insurance, etc.).

Sadly, the United States also has many features that adversely affect the market for healthcare services. Insurers operate in an environment where product differentiation is not only allowed, it has almost become a marketing necessity for each carrier since each must piece together a package of benefits that it can provide at a competitive price. Each carrier simply must have a product line that it can afford to sell. Consequently, purchasers of health insurance must sort through a dizzying array of benefit packages hoping to find a suitable policy at a suitable price. Previous discussion in Chapter Eight has addressed the benefits of a uniform MBBP.

Even though a uniform MBBP might decrease the degree of product differentiation in the health insurance market, it is unrealistic to imagine that product differentiation will completely disappear. Medical expertise will continue to vary by region and institution, and expert specialty care will probably always command a higher fee. Some variety associated with the delivery of MBBP is to be expected.

Another feature of the U.S. health insurance market is price differentiation. Simply put, price differentiation means that even with similar health risks, different purchasers of the exact same insurance coverage may pay different prices; the critical determinant of price being the negotiating capacity of the purchasers.[40]

Effects of Price Differentiation

Both product differentiation and price differentiation are widely practiced outside health insurance markets. Vendors in many markets routinely employ price differentiation to increase profits. With price differentiation a company can generate the same revenues as it could at competitive market prices, but can charge higher prices to some and can save money by limiting production.

Presently, insurers operate in a market environment where price differentiation is commonplace. Large groups and corporations can insure themselves at lower costs because they have lower administrative costs and spread costs over larger populations; they can therefore negotiate the price of premiums from a position of advantage. Smaller organizations and individuals with lesser bargaining power pay higher insurance costs. And an individual with pre-existing medical conditions may actually be priced out of the health insurance market.

Product differentiation and price differentiation have become necessary tools for survival in the current risk-rated environment of the U.S. health insurance market. Both the insured and the uninsured populations have paid for this circumstance. The insured have paid in dollars, and the uninsured have paid in terms of health.

The effects of price differentiation on market dynamics can be illustrated with a Price/Quantity curve. In Figure 2, under current circumstances, health insurance carriers sell insurance under conditions of price differentiation. In the current situation P1 is the lowest negotiable price and P1' is the highest price successfully charged. At P1/Q1 insurers may limit sales to low risk individuals and will have revenues equal to the entire area left of Q1, including the triangular area above P1. In this situation, insurees with limited bargaining power must pay more than P1 for health insurance; they pay a premium closer to P1' — at the high end of the negotiable price range.

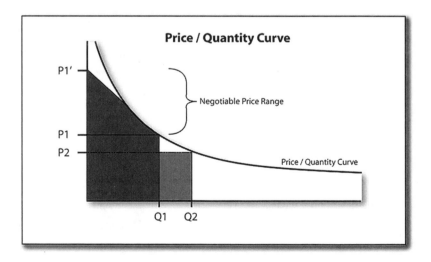

Figure 2. Current Price/Quantity Curve

Under conditions of universal enrollment without price differentiation, however, the market price changes. In a price competitive market insurers will have revenues equal to the <u>enclosed</u> <u>rectangular</u> area left of Q2. Without price differentiation, P2 becomes the market price for everyone! No one pays at P1'.

Policy Goals

The primary goal of a universal healthcare policy is, of course, universal coverage; a secondary goal is to achieve this at a lower market price. And if policy makers impose regulations on insurers supportive of the essential conditions for successful distribution of goods in a competitive market (namely uniformity of product, community ratings, and guaranteed issue), a lower price, P2, may be attainable. In any case, insurers will now be competing on price, convenience, service, and reputation and not on the ability to identify insurees' potential health risks.

Two factors change the dynamics of health insurance markets when insurance becomes mandatory and the market becomes price competitive:

- *the population to be insured increases, thus shifting the entire demand curve to the right, and*
- *the marginal cost of insuring a new client becomes lower.*

Both changes are favorable to insurers.

Shift in Demand

The first of these changes is a change in the quantity demanded. Demand shifts to the right as enrollment increases from Q1 to Q2, and the demand curve now becomes vertical, or as economists would say, "inelastic." Both the shift to the right and the change to a vertical position are the result of mandatory or default enrollment. The shift to the right reflects the inclusion into the market of that 15% of the U.S. population who are currently uninsured, and the vertical alignment reflects the fact that enrollment is now mandatory — the entire population is now enrolled. This new Q2 allows for increased revenues in a competitive environment under conditions of community ratings.

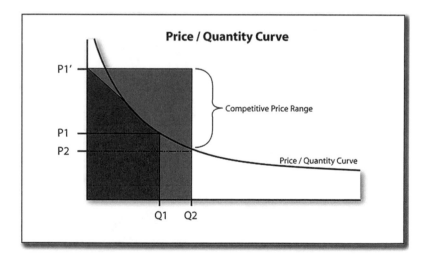

Figure 3. Price/Quantity Curve after Shift in Demand

Under these conditions, a monopoly could price premiums at P1', but even the most efficient GHI could not provide healthcare benefits at a price lower than P2, thus generating the competitive price range. Under these circumstances, if any insurer priced a healthcare premium below P1, all insurers would have to meet or beat that price to remain in the market. An example of this scenario is further discussed in Chapter Twelve where a universal healthcare model is proposed.

Decreased Marginal Costs

The second change, a decrease in marginal costs, reflects reduced risk when accepting the incremental insuree under the market conditions associated with mandatory enrollment. This occurs because the uninsured are largely healthy workers and because mandatory health insurance will include not only the high-risk, but also the low-risk individuals in the funding pool. Under the present market conditions where health insurance is risk rated, and not mandatory, the uninsured naturally divide themselves into two groups, those who perceive themselves to have low risk of disease, and those who perceive themselves to have increased risk of disease.

Those who perceive that they have lower risk do not seek health insurance, but those who perceive that they do have increased risk do seek health insurance. It is the group of potential insurees with increased risk who seek health insurance and who generate high marginal costs (and who persuade insurers to differentiate price based on risk). But when the healthy portion of the uninsured are included in the insurance pool, a consequence of mandatory insurance, the marginal cost falls, reflecting the reduced incremental costs that accompany their inclusion.

Discussion

The achievement of P2, the lowest feasible competitive price for health insurance — and a reduction in price below P1 — implies that under a competitive market system such as this, improved efficiencies in health insurance management and in healthcare delivery are possible. Certainly, when one considers the success of the countries of the OECD, attainment of this goal appears very realistic. In 2003, even the next least efficient system, the Swiss system where 100% of the population is privately insured, had per capita healthcare costs of approximately US$3,200 compared to per capita costs of $4,500 in the U.S. In other words, the Swiss spent 29% less per capita on healthcare than the U.S.!

> Even the next least efficient system in the world, the Swiss system, where 100% of the population is privately insured, has per capita healthcare costs 29% less than the U.S.

Application of this model implies an understanding of two conditions. First, it must be remembered that the cost of issuing a health insurance policy is not simply the cost of selling another piece of paper titled "Health Insurance." Rather the entire cost of providing medical services to the newly insured client must be considered. The average cost of providing those medical services is the cost for which insurers must prepare and is the cost of a health insurance premium under conditions of community ratings. Although it is tempting to imagine that the per capita costs of will drop sharply in a market driven environment (one might be tempted to imagine — incorrectly — that it cannot cost all that much to issue another insurance policy), there will surely be a cost for health insurance below which insurers cannot assure coverage of all desired healthcare benefits. Below that price, access to certain services must be limited, either through intentional exclusion of some services or through soft rationing by limiting infrastructure and manpower and establishing waiting lists. The market price of health insurance cannot drop forever. This is illustrated by the failure of the Price/Quantity curve to approach zero.

Second, the shift to the right of the Quantity can only occur freely when there is sufficient capacity in the healthcare system to accommodate the increase in utilization that will occur when those presently uninsured are provided with access to healthcare benefits. If there is insufficient capacity in the system when healthcare coverage is made mandatory, there will either be price increases in both medical services and health insurance premiums, or there will be "soft rationing" resulting from the new demand for services. In a competitive market environment, however, it is reasonable to anticipate that the following market mechanisms will assure sufficient capacity in the healthcare system:

- *The increase in demand will be small enough that present capacity will be sufficient. This may be expected if the following assumptions hold:*

  - *92% of the uninsured enjoy "good," "very good," or "excellent" health (only 8% claim their health is less than "good").*

  - *15% of the total population is uninsured.*

  - *Therefore, the proportion of the total population that is presently both uninsured and also claims that its health is less than "good" is quite small, about 1.2% (15% x 8% = 1.2%).*

  - *Even if 100% of these people seek medical care, the present healthcare capacity should surely accommodate an additional 1.2% increase in demand for services. And even if the increased demand for medical care is three times that amount, there is still only an increase in total utilization of 3.6%.*

- *Newly discovered efficiencies in the system will offset any increased demand for services. There are estimates of billions of dollars of potential savings by implementing certain standards for electronic data, such as:*

  - *Uniform medical records systems*

  - *Uniform billing systems*

  - *Shared medical records*

  - *Uniform accounting methods*

- *A more competitive environment will drive increased efficiency in utilization of present resources.*

- *As prices begin to rise, new providers will enter the market and prices will return to competitive levels.*

Any or all of the above mechanisms suggest that the shift in Quantity may freely occur.

Conclusion

In this model, with even a minimal decrease in the market price for health insurance below the lowest negotiable price (P1), there will be cost savings for small businesses and individual buyers of insurance — and potentially for some large purchasers of insurance. Additionally, the United States will have achieved universal healthcare and retained the benefits of a dynamic market.

The effects of this model represent dramatic changes for the U.S. healthcare market, but dramatic changes are warranted.

Selvoy M. Fillerup, MD, MSPH, FACS

CHAPTER TEN

Sorry, Mister, you can't get there from here!

As stated previously, the goals of any universal healthcare policy are universal enrollment (access) and cost containment (solvency). Policy makers worry that universal enrollment will drastically increase healthcare costs. Ironically, mandatory universal enrollment in healthcare contributes to lower per capita healthcare costs by limiting the risks and costs associated with risk-oriented insurance models — or so it would seem from the OECD experience. Without universal enrollment the United States may never even come close to cost containment!

Adverse selection, a factor in any risk-mitigation model, has a large effect on costs. But in the arena of health insurance, the costs associated with adverse selection largely disappear under universal enrollment, and universal enrollment may change the entire business model for health insurance from a risk-mitigation model to a cost redistribution model and truly bring healthcare costs in line with costs in other industrialized nations.

Adverse Selection

The following description of adverse selection is pertinent to health insurance:

> *"People who buy insurance often have a better idea of the risks they face than do the sellers of insurance. People who know that they face large risks are more likely to buy insurance than people who face small risks. Insurance companies try to minimize the problem that only the people with big risks will buy their product, which is the problem of adverse selection, by trying to measure risk and to adjust prices they charge for this risk. Thus, life insurance companies require medical examinations and will refuse policies to people who have terminal illnesses, and automobile insurance companies charge much more to people with a conviction for drunk driving." (Robert Schenk, Insurance, web page)* [44]

Adverse selection was initially described by the Nobel Prize winning economist George A. Akerlof, who noted that when a buyer had insufficient information about the product he or she was buying, the seller could sell inferior goods at elevated prices. This places the buyer at risk–the risk of "adversely selecting" an inferior good at a price higher than its true value.

In the insurance industry the tables are turned. It is the seller of the insurance policy who must beware. The buyer of the policy may withhold health related information (known only to the buyer) from the insurer, thus placing the insurer at risk for paying unexpected health related costs in excess of anticipated collectible premiums. The insurance company has "adversely selected" a high-risk client.

In the field of health insurance, "adverse selection" has come to refer the entire concept of clients buying health insurance only when they anticipate using medical services. To mitigate the financial risk associated with adverse selection, insurers "price differentiate"; they charge higher premiums to clients with increased healthcare risks or higher administrative costs.

Remember that under present market conditions in the United States, where health insurance is risk-rated and not mandatory, the uninsured, or at least that portion who could afford health insurance, naturally divide themselves into two groups: those who perceive themselves to have low risk of disease, and those who perceive themselves to have increased risk of disease.

Those who perceive that they have lower risk <u>do not seek</u> health insurance, but those who perceive that they do have increased risk <u>do seek</u> health insurance. It is the group of potential insurees with increased risk, who seek health insurance, who generate high marginal costs (and who persuade insurers to differentiate insurance products and prices based on risk).

The Pool of Uninsured Contribute to Adverse Selection

Although the number of uninsured remains relatively constant, every year — indeed every month — some individuals lose their health insurance coverage and some individuals become insured. Estimates by the U.S. Census Bureau Survey of Income and Program Participation suggest that on average, about 15% of the United States population is uninsured at any time, and that about 90% of Americans have health insurance for at least one month of the year.[45]

At first, one might assume that the problem of the uninsured is not really so large after all; only about 10% of the population remains uninsured for an entire year. However, over a 32-month period of time, one in four Americans (25%) will be without health insurance for at least one month.[46] This pool of uninsured is the real problem.

This large pool of potential insurees generates adverse selection and thereby justifies the practices of price and product differentiation. A tremendously large number of insurance seekers, 25% of the United States' population, rotate through the uninsured population each year. Naturally, insurers want to protect themselves against insuring the high-risk individuals who become insured. It makes no difference to the new insurer whether these are people who have been uninsured for a long period of time or have only recently become uninsured. It will cost the new insurer the same amount to provide them with medical services.

Insurers never know who will decide that their health status is such that they need health insurance or when they will do so. When these people do decide they need health insurance, insurers face the risk that medical expenses will exceed the amount that will be collected in premiums. They face the problem called adverse selection.

It is no surprise then that insurers are more willing to insure families that receive insurance as an employment benefit. These are people with new jobs who want to go to work, whereas the family that purchases health insurance privately may simply be applying for health insurance based on the perceived need for medical care.

The number of newly insured each year is substantial. Because the newly insured have not been paying into the new insurance companies' insurance funds, the money to provide for their care must come from those who have already paid into that fund. In this manner the "long-term insured" subsidize the "short-term insured," and the insurance company is merely keeping the books (for a fee, of course). The problem of adverse selection thus becomes the problem and expense of the long-term insured population.

> The "long-term insured" subsidize the "short-term insured" and the insurance company is merely keeping the books (for a fee, of course).

In this regard, the cost of adverse selection is the cost of medical care for the newly insured plus administrative costs, including underwriting expenses, to redistribute the costs of the "short-term insured" among the "long-term insured."

The exact portion of total healthcare costs directly attributable to adverse selection may not be readily identifiable, and it would be foolish to assume that adverse selection was the sole cause of the difference in healthcare costs between the United States and other nations; but the expense of price differentiation associated with adverse selection does not exist among countries with universal healthcare because in nations with universal healthcare there is no pool of uninsured.

The True Cost of the Absence of Universal Enrollment

The root cause for price and product differentiation — justified by adverse selection — is the absence of universal enrollment. Adverse selection may be the engine that sustains price differentiation and high insurance costs, but the fuel for that engine is the absence of a universal enrollment policy.

Figure 4, shown previously in Chapter Nine and shown again below, represents a production (price and quantity) curve for health insurance. In this figure Q1 represents the current level of health insurance enrollment. at a given level of care. P1 represents the lowest negotiable premium for health insurance and P1' represents the highest premium an insurer can successfully charge. Total insurance revenues are shown as the darkly shaded area left of Q1, including revenues derived through the practice of price differentiation (represented by the triangular area left of Q1 and above P1). Q2 would represent the number enrolled in healthcare plans if there were a national policy enforcing universal enrollment. The average price of health insurance falls between P1 and P1'. P2 would be the market price for healthcare under conditions of universal enrollment and community rating — conditions that exist in nations with universal healthcare.

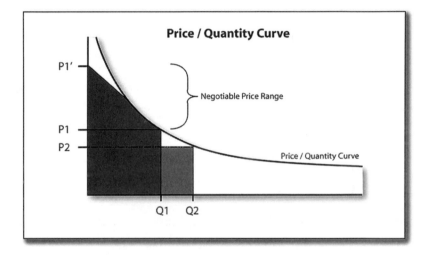

Figure 4: Current Price/Quantity Curve

Although high health insurance prices are the result of price differentiation, and price differentiation is sustained by adverse selection, the true cost to consumers of health insurance in this situation is not due to adverse selection or price differentiation. The true cost to consumers is the inability of the present United

States system to reach the P2/Q2 equilibrium state. This is the equilibrium state that nations with universal enrollment have already attained and arguably contributes to lower overall healthcare costs.

Unless universal enrollment is achieved (Q2), truly lower insurance costs (P2) cannot be achieved. It is the absence of a universal enrollment policy that maintains a population of insurance seekers rotating through the uninsured population pool as if through a revolving door, fueling adverse selection and sustaining price differentiation.

Conclusion

The risk associated with adverse selection, and the justification by insurers to practice price differentiation, begins with the absence of a healthcare policy that mandates universal enrollment and fosters a communal cost-sharing model for health insurance. Private health insurance can and does perform this function in other countries.[11] But healthcare systems cannot reach P2 without universal enrollment.[47]

Only a national policy of universal enrollment will contribute to lower health insurance costs by eliminating the costs associated with adverse selection. This will allow the United States health insurance market to eliminate the practice of price differentiation and thereby attain the same market equilibrium already attained by other nations.

CHAPTER ELEVEN

Secondary Benefits

"I am not an advocate for frequent changes in laws and constitutions, but laws and institutions must go hand in hand with the progress of the human mind. As that becomes more developed, more enlightened, as new discoveries are made, new truths discovered and manners and opinions change, institutions must advance also to keep pace with the times. We might as well require a man to wear still the same coat which fitted him when a boy as civilized society to remain forever under the regimen of their barbarous ancestors."

Thomas Jefferson, (displayed in the rotunda of the Jefferson memorial)

Healthcare has become a chronic crisis in the United States. Because of the sophistication and expense associated with modern medical services, independent payment for medical care has become impossible. The days of paying for medical care with a couple of chickens and an apple pie are gone. Forever.

In response to this reality, private insurance and health management cooperatives evolved in the mid twentieth century. There have been efforts by various administrations to bring the entire population under a U.S. government managed healthcare system, but these efforts have failed.

The result is a collage of healthcare organizations — some governmental, some private, some for profit, some not-for-profit — to share in the task of providing healthcare to U.S. citizens. But no cohesive healthcare policy has evolved. Certainly no <u>universal</u> healthcare policy has evolved, and a substantial portion of the U.S. population, 15%, remains without healthcare coverage — the "uninsured." The United States has relied increasingly on generosity from a loose coalition of donors, providers, and hospitals — a so-called "safety net" — to provide healthcare to this segment of the population. The safety net is wearing thin.

Aside from direct donations to assist those without access to health insurance, this safety net relies heavily on the practice of "cost-shifting" to finance medical services for the uninsured. Both private insurers and government (through Medicare) at one time paid sufficiently high prices for the medical services of their patients that cost-shifting was tolerated. In a sense, but obviously without any stated policy to do so, hospitals and physician were expected to cost-shift in order to cover the medical needs of those who could not afford health insurance or who did not qualify for government healthcare benefits. But cost-shifting is no longer an efficient or palatable means of distributing healthcare costs; government has determined that Medicare and

Medicaid should cover only the medical costs of their enrolled populations — and no more!

Health insurance companies have followed this practice of paying only as much as necessary for medical services. They now negotiate fees to their lowest achievable levels, leaving no extra funds on the table for providers to apply to cost-shifting. The so-called safety net, in the absence of funds available for the purpose of cost-shifting, is slipping into a position of diminished capacity in regard to providing for the uninsured. The diminished capacity of the safety net indirectly affects the entire population.

The high cost of health insurance in the United States has created a number of economic and social problems. It has contributed to a greater number of under-insured and uninsured individuals living in the United States, and forced people to either ration or not purchase the care they need.[50]

As mentioned earlier, both from a sense of moral obligation and for reasons of social and financial stability, previous administrations have attempted to institute systems of universal healthcare in the United States. State and national leaders have understood that the financial and social benefits of universal healthcare outweigh any benefit of the status quo; the lack of universal healthcare hampers the delivery of healthcare services at multiple levels.[51] It is the purpose of this chapter to review at least some of the secondary economic and social benefits that will almost certainly accompany implementation of a universal healthcare policy.

Benefits Associated with Universal Healthcare.

1. The simplest and the first benefit of universal healthcare is the obvious benefit: the nation will enjoy improved health. This is particularly true for those who otherwise would have no healthcare coverage. Among OECD countries, comparative health status statistics related to longevity strongly suggest that universal health programs prolong life and increase the quality of life compared to the United States — and do so at a lower per capita cost and a lower percentage of GDP.[19]

2. Among the associated macro-economic benefits of universal healthcare is increased workforce productivity. It seems only too obvious that this would be true; it occurs in two ways. First, healthy individuals are well enough to work and be productive and are available to teach and train; unhealthy individuals are either not available for work or are not as productive when they are at work as confirmed by measurements of lost productivity and lost wages.[52-61]

Second, sickness and disease are burdens that siphon resources away from other profitable endeavors. The direct costs of medical treatments represent opportunity costs; the cost of caring for an ill population reduces resources that would otherwise be used to finance schools or highways or support other economic development. (An extreme example of this is the cost of treating malaria in Africa. The direct and indirect costs of treating between 300 million and 500 million cases of malaria per year or over a million cases per day has immeasurably hampered economic development in tropical Africa for decades.[62])

3. The same benefits occur on a micro-economic scale. Ill breadwinners are less productive and may not be able to afford to pay for education, housing or a healthy diet for themselves or for a family. They may not even be able to provide basic nurturing. Likewise, a family that must independently shoulder the burdens of paying the medical expenses of one ill child may not be able to afford educational opportunities for other children.

4. Subtle social discrimination on the part of the healthcare industry would end; no person would be denied healthcare coverage because of race, genetic conditions, or for pre-existing conditions. Under current conditions, it is possible for such persons to be charged prohibitively high premiums for health insurance if they have a known medical condition. Caught in this situation, many people forego health insurance citing prohibitive cost as the reason. Without healthcare coverage, people do not seek routine healthcare and do not receive preventive care. The subsequent underutilization of primary and preventive care results in untreated health problems, late diagnoses of cancers, and other chronic illnesses resulting in loss of physical function in many cases. But if healthcare were universal, those who most need healthcare would be able to receive it without discrimination.

5. Health insurance has been shown to affect utilization and indirectly affect the costs of medical care. Both the costs and benefits associated with extending

health insurance coverage depend on the extent to and manner in which health insurance affects the utilization of medical services. Overall, health insurance status has significant effects on all types of utilization. Insurance coverage increases outpatient utilization and is associated with an increased receipt of preventive care. Furthermore, there is some evidence that insurance coverage reduces ambulatory care sensitive hospital admissions.[63]

6. Current federal regulations indirectly encourage the uninsured to use the most expensive source of medical care available, the emergency room, as their main source of medical care. Those presently uninsured would be able to use a primary care provider as their main source of care. Primary care is less expensive than emergency care.

> Current federal regulations indirectly encourage he uninsured to use the most expensive source of medical care available — the emergency room.

7. Timely treatment of illness is generally less expensive than management of the complications associated with late treatment. Saving would occur when needy patients received earlier and less costly primary care rather than waiting until their diseases become so advanced that they seek expensive tertiary care.

8. There will be indirect economic benefits to those already insured. If everyone had some form of health insurance, hospitals could stop the practice of cost-shifting. Unnecessary emergency care must be paid for with funds from those who do pay (cost-shifting) or from

charities. If hospitals and providers are to provide free emergency room care, they must engage in cost-shifting. Cost-shifting requires that paying patients — those already insured — must pay amounts in excess of the true cost of their medical care. But under a system of universal healthcare, the necessity to engage in the practice of cost-shifting would almost disappear, thus opening the opportunity to lower the cost of individual health insurance.

9. All patients could be given therapeutic treatment. Hospital emergency rooms are required only to provide emergency care sufficient to stabilize a patient, but not to provide curative therapy. If universal healthcare were implemented, hospitals could stop turning away needy patients who needed curative care; hospitals would be paid for all medical services.

10. Inner city hospitals would become less dependent on tax revenues, charities, and cost-shifting to remain solvent. Emergency rooms could focus on emergency medical services rather than providing outpatient clinical services in an expensive setting and could reallocate resources accordingly. Donations presently used to fund the total costs of much charity healthcare could be used to cover deductibles and co-payments for charity cases, and the balance could be made available for research, education, or additional infrastructure.

11. Bankruptcies related to medical expenses would decrease; families would no longer risk bankruptcy by paying healthcare costs for ill family members. Accumulated medical debt is disproportionate to the U.S. median annual gross income, and in one study, medical

debt accounted for at least 25% of all personal bankruptcies.[50]

12. One very important social and economic benefit that should not be underestimated is the increased mobility of the workforce that would follow implementation of universal healthcare. Increased productivity of the workforce would be the direct result of a mobile workforce; employers would be able to match job opportunities to employees' skills, thereby increasing productivity.

As previously stated, workers would be free to seek other rewarding employment without fear of losing healthcare benefits. With universally available healthcare benefits, a worker in Minneapolis could accept new employment in Atlanta knowing that healthcare benefits would be available. Employers could compete for productive workers without concerns about matching health insurance benefits.

13. There would be additional health benefits to those already insured if the entire population was insured. In the absence of universal healthcare, if an infectious epidemic were to occur, the uninsured population would be slow to seek treatment and become a reservoir of untreated disease with the potential of infecting the remaining population. Every one of us would benefit if all of us had access to early treatment for contagious diseases.

14. Much of the lost productivity surrounding labor negotiations could be averted if universal healthcare was implemented. Speaking of a grocery workers strike in 2004, Greg Denier, assistant to the international

president of the UFCW, said the strike "would not have occurred if we had a system of universal healthcare coverage. All of our strikes in the past decade have occurred because of the absence of universal healthcare."

Moreover, universal health coverage would have "a profound effect" not just on the supermarket industry but "on nearly all collective bargaining," according to lawyer Harry Burton, representing Safeway and Giant Food (2004). Nonunion companies "virtually never" provide healthcare of the same quality as that provided by unionized competitors, thus creating "a vast disparity in costs." Universal healthcare would narrow the wide gap in operating costs between the unionized chains and nonunion competitors.

15. Part-time and temporary employees might soon be offered full-time employment if their employers had to contribute to their healthcare benefits anyway. Currently, many persons are only given part-time employment so that employers do not have to contribute to health insurance costs, but if employers had to contribute toward healthcare benefits regardless of full or part-time status of employees, the country might realize increased full-time employment rates, thereby increasing national productivity. If more people became full-time employees, they would be better able to afford their premiums.

16. The country might find that fewer people require welfare benefits. If unemployed heads-of-household did not fear losing healthcare benefits by becoming employed, more of them might seek employment.

17. Insurance companies might take a more active interest in public health if preventive medical practices influenced profitability; certainly earlier detection of cancer lowers treatment costs and saves lives, and earlier intervention in diabetes lowers the cost of chronic care and reduces morbidity. Conceivably, insurance companies could reduce expenditures if such chronic conditions were managed earlier and might be motivated to do so if they had to enroll all who applied.

18. Industry might be more aggressive in promoting technologies proven to lower healthcare costs. There might be an impetus to share and secure medical records electronically if that information could not be used to discriminate against those with known medical conditions. The savings from this effort alone has been estimated to save hundreds of millions of dollars.

Conclusion

The current opportunities to improve health and reduce the costs of healthcare require that serious consideration be given to a national healthcare policy, including universal healthcare. Aside from the obvious initial health benefits to those who are presently uninsured, there are many secondary economic benefits to universal healthcare. Universal healthcare would affect workers and the economy in many ways and would open the door to opportunities for savings in operating and administrative costs as well.

CHAPTER TWELVE

Keep It Simple

The following pages contain a proposal for a multi-payor universal healthcare system. The details of such a model are much less important than the foundation upon which it is built. The details should be flexible; the model itself should be dynamic. In fact, it must be dynamic if it is to survive. One might think of it as similar to a building; move a wall, move a window, or change the heating system, so long as the foundation is firm, the building will stand.

Begin with a Policy

There must first be a healthcare policy and a plan to accomplish that policy with the stated intent of providing universal healthcare.

As previously stated, citizens must assign the role of policy maker to government; once given that role, government has certain tasks to perform. Among these tasks is the decision regarding the basic direction of policy — the "path" that the healthcare system will follow. (Recently, the journal <u>Healthcare Politics, Policy and Law</u> devoted an entire issue to the long term effects of "path dependency."[1] It is no wonder that no one seems willing to adopt a policy without a vision of where that path will lead.)

Will the path follow the route of a single-payor system or a competitive multi-payor system?

Other basic decisions deal with the roles of GHI and PHI. Will there be only GHI, or only PHI, or both? And if both, there must be complementary roles for both. What will be the role of GHI? Of PHI? How, exactly, will they complement one another?

Government must reserve certain powers to itself and must assign specific responsibilities to GHI. Government may allow PHI certain privileges and must impose upon PHI certain constraints in order to accomplish its policy goals, including access and solvency for the healthcare system.

Other nations have built models that succeed, and so can the United States.

The Minimum Basic Benefits Package

The task falls to legislative government to determine the level of care in a minimum basic benefits package (MBBP). (What a marvelous debate this will be! Every interest group in healthcare will be there! The beginnings should be modest; the program will be much more difficult to shrink than to grow.)

Vulnerable Populations

Government must define vulnerable populations and must determine whether GHI will cover only specific vulnerable populations (as it presently does) or if GHI will cover the entire population. If government elects to cover the entire population, it must then decide whether to provide a high level of coverage, as has been done in Canada, the United Kingdom and Scandinavia, or coverage only to a limited degree, as has been done in France.

If the choice is for GHI to cover only some "vulnerable" portion of the population, then who shall they be? In the case of the Netherlands, the decision was made to cover the two-thirds of the population with the lowest income. In Japan GHI covers the agricultural sector, the self-employed, and the elderly. The United States has already decided that GHI will cover the poor and elderly. (The wisdom in any of these choices may be debated, but not here.) Keep in mind that by deciding which portion of the population will be covered by GHI, government also decides which portion will be covered by PHI — or not at all!

In all countries compromises have been made to accommodate the needs of the chronically ill and the poor. In Switzerland and Germany insurance companies apply to a special government fund to subsidize insurance for the chronically ill. In the Netherlands and in Japan the very ill are removed from the GHI insurance pool that insures workers and other retirees but are insured through a special fund. In France, where basic health needs are covered for everyone, and private "complementary" insurance covers 86% of the population for the balance of their costs, the government purchases complementary insurance for those who otherwise could never afford it.

In the U.S., Medicaid and SCHIPS are already in place to care for the poor and for uninsured children, and Medicare covers the elderly. The decision to continue or alter these programs will remain in the healthcare debate.

The Revenue Stream

Government must establish a revenue stream in order to finance its selected healthcare activities. Several methods have been discussed already. One model is to have an income-based (shared between employer and employee) revenue stream. In Japan, this is done by literally thousands of insurance cooperatives; the health cooperatives first negotiate services and fees with providers and then simply pass those estimated costs to their members — the employers and employees — to be shared equally between them based on wage scales.

Another method is to have a tax-based revenue system. Some European systems use this method, employing a consumption-based sales tax to fund social services. In any tax-based revenue system, revenues are linked to the political will to increase taxes and not to the demand for medical services.

Another option is the production based Solidarity system. But remember that tax-based methods and the Solidarity system have the disadvantage of yielding a fixed amount of revenue that must then be budgeted to cover GHI services. When the funds run out, some form of soft rationing may be anticipated.

Countries with high percentages of the population covered by PHI rely on insurance companies to spread the costs of medical services across the population. Such systems have little or no soft rationing — no prolonged waiting times for elective medical services; revenues are more directly linked to demands for medical services. Countries with large markets for PHI rely on competition to contain the costs of both premiums and services, but in these countries it is important to have regulations that preserve a normal market environment.

Expenditures

Government must also decide how it will pay its providers; it must establish a payment system and determine the level of payment for services. In many healthcare systems, GHI simply sets fees. In other systems, fees are negotiated. In the United States, providers for GHI are still paid on a fee-for-service method modified by Diagnosis Related Groups (DRGs) and Relative Value Scales (RVS).

Government must also decide whether the money follows the patient or follows the system. In the United Kingdom, healthcare is not thought of as a menu of individual medical services, but as an entire set of social services for which providers are paid for their availability (time) and the wellness of their assigned populations (outcomes). As such, the money follows the services and the system rather than the individual patient.

The Relationship Between GHI and PHI

Finally the government must determine the role of PHI and the relationship between GHI and PHI. Government retains the obligation to protect public interests as defined by healthcare policy and must enact and enforce regulations such that health insurance is available at a competitive market price. Insurance companies in other countries with other regulatory environments have managed to continue doing business when uniform policies have been mandatory, when community ratings have been enforced, and when issue is guaranteed.

> Government retains the obligation to protect public interests as defined by healthcare policy and must enact and enforce regulations such that health insurance is available at a competitive market price

Basic Elements of a Multi-payor Universal Healthcare Model

The policy tools necessary to build a multi-payor universal healthcare system in the United States have been reviewed. The role of government has been reviewed, including the responsibility to establish a regulated market environment with a uniform MBBP. The effects of a uniform health insurance policy have been demonstrated in several OECD countries. The effects of community ratings and guaranteed issue have been described, including their relative success in some of the countries where they have been enforced. However, in the U.S. where such measures are not in place, the poor and the ill are compelled to accept lower levels of coverage, or higher health insurance premiums, or higher deductibles and co-pays, or to go without insurance.

Parameters of Policy

This model begins with the intent to establish a policy. Initially, government must mandate that everyone will be insured. Government must then foster an environment conducive to competition based on price, convenience, amenities, and reputation rather than on administrative costs or risk. There must be a market with a sufficiently large number of insurers to promote competition. In order for insurers to compete based on price, they must be required to offer the same minimum basic benefits policy, and they must be required to sell it to any who apply to purchase it.

Such a policy, based on these fundamentals and unique to the United States, can succeed.

The following are the elements of a proposed policy in outline form.

- *Government will determine the parameters of the MBBP.*
- *The same MBBP will apply to both GHI and PHI.*
- *The same MBBP is offered*
    - *to the employees of large employers.*

- *to employees of small employers.*
- *temporary and part-time employees.*
- *individual insurance purchasers.*
- *to those currently uninsured as well as those enrolled in GHI.*
- *Health insurance will be mandatory.*
- *Health insurance will be offered under conditions of*
  - *Community ratings.*
  - *Guaranteed issue.*
- *There are no barriers to switching between carriers.*
  - *Regulations must favor a substantial number of carriers.*
  - *Bundling of benefits packages is prohibited.*
- *Employees of large corporations must choose PHI.*
  - *Large corporations are defined as having more than 500 employees.*
  - *GHI will not accept individuals from this market.*
- *All others (small employers, the privately insured, and the uninsured) may choose either GHI or PHI.*
- *GHI will cover vulnerable populations.*
  - *Currently defined as Medicare, Medicaid, the military and others.*
  - *GHI insures all who are unable or unwilling to purchase PHI.*
  - *GHI collects premiums (through the tax system) from all non-vulnerable enrollees.*
    - *This premium is structured in such a way that it is not overly comfortable for non-vulnerable populations to elect GHI.*
    - *low income or unemployed GHI enrollees may receive other tax credits, but are still charged a healthcare premium.*

- *Employers and employees share the cost of health insurance (including all full-time, part-time and temporary employees).*

- *PHI competes in all markets except Medicare, Medicaid and the military.*

Defining Populations and the Complementary Roles of GHI and PHI

In the report *Income, Poverty, and Health Insurance Coverage in the United States: 2003,*[3] the uninsured population is estimated at 13.7% of the population, and GHI covers an estimated at 29.6% of the population (Medicare, Medicaid, the military and others). This same report estimates that 69.6% of the population has private health insurance, 9.2% is obtained privately and 60.4% is obtained through employment. Other estimates differ. (The numbers in this report add up to greater than 100% suggesting that some individuals have more than one source of cover, but for the purposes of this discussion, these numbers are fine.)

Additionally, the Small Business Administration estimates that half of all employees work in businesses with fewer than 500 employees.[48,49] This estimate is used to divide the employment-based PHI market into two equal segments, each consisting of about 30.2% of the population. From these estimates, the following chart showing insurance by type has been derived.

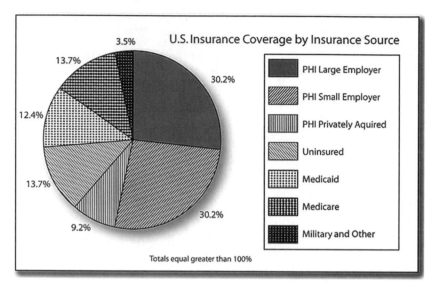

Figure 5: Insurance Coverage by Insurance Source

Shown in a different format, insurance by type looks like this:

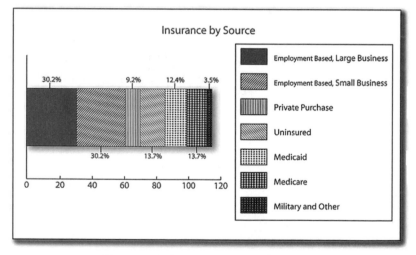

Figure 6: Insurance by Source

Among the parameters for a universal healthcare system, GHI is designated to care for previously defined vulnerable populations: Medicare, Medicaid, and the military. The three areas at the right of the bar chart represent the populations covered by GHI.

It is also a condition of this model that GHI will not offer its services to large businesses — those with more than 500 employees. The large business segment of the health insurance market will be reserved to PHI. GHI will not seek to insure that segment of the market, and the employees of large corporations may not apply to GHI for health insurance coverage. This will preserve to PHI a market and a population of working enrollees whose health status is already understood by PHI.

The remaining segments of the market, shown in the central segment of the bar, the employees of small businesses, the privately insured, and the uninsured, would then be allowed to choose enrollment in either PHI or GHI. PHI and GHI would essentially compete for these sectors of the market (just as package delivery services like FedEx and UPS compete with the U.S. Postal Service). All full-time employees of small businesses, all part-time and temporary employees, the self-employed, and the uninsured would then have health insurance through either PHI or through GHI. Any who failed to enroll in PHI would, by default, be enrolled in GHI.

Vulnerable and Non-Vulnerable Populations

Finally, as discussed in Chapter Eight, it should not be overly comfortable for non-vulnerable populations to enroll in GHI if the true policy goal is to alleviate GHI of the responsibility of administering healthcare coverage to non-vulnerable populations.

For non-vulnerable populations enrolled in GHI, it should be the responsibility of government to charge a premium sufficient to cover the costs of insurance. Admittedly, this will look like a tax, and be collected like a tax, but it should in all actuality be an insurance premium. There may be some who will object to this position, claiming that the working poor require special consideration, but in reality this is simply a matter of clarifying the distinction between vulnerable and non-vulnerable populations.

Those who are poor enough to be enrolled in Medicaid should be enrolled in Medicaid — this is where those who are poor enough to be included among "vulnerable populations" receive healthcare benefits. If criteria for enrollment in Medicaid need to be expanded to include an additional 2 or 3% of the population, or if some in-between status — or quasi-vulnerable status — needs to be defined for the working poor, those problems can be solved. Options such as Earned Income Tax credits have already been mentioned.

But non-vulnerable populations, which account for the huge majority of the uninsured, have the capacity to pay toward their own healthcare.

The "Shared Market"

Admittedly, under such a model, government policy will ultimately determine the parameters of competition and the market share of PHI. PHI is already a highly regulated industry, and government could possibly set the terms of competition such that GHI had the entire market to itself. In such an alternate scenario, if the policy goal is to achieve the lowest possible price for healthcare services, GHI may offer a premium priced as low as it deems feasible, thus compelling PHI to meet or beat that low price in order to have any business whatsoever in this market segment.

But the point of having PHI as a participant in a universal healthcare policy is to employ the unique features of PHI that make it successful at administering the costs of medical care across populations — specifically, to use PHI as a source of funding for infrastructure and technology, to exploit the responsiveness of PHI to market demands, to relieve GHI of certain costs and case loads, to utilize the capacity of PHI to devise and implement efficient management practices, and of course, to distribute costs and remain solvent.

There will almost certainly be some proportion of the shared population enrolled in GHI. There will always be those who, for philosophic reasons, prefer GHI over PHI, and vice-versa, just as there are many who advocate single-payor systems and often cite the efficiency of governments to contain administrative costs as justification for that opinion. And there will almost certainly be a segment of the population who simply do not act, or are unwilling to seek PHI and thus elect GHI. And, yes, government could stack the deck in such a manner that PHI could not compete for these market segments, although that would defeat the point of sharing this market. But there is little doubt in my mind that PHI can successfully compete with GHI for the majority of this shared market. Furthermore, PHI will likely lobby for constraints on GHI such that citizens have an incentive to enroll in PHI.

Preserving a Dynamic System

Ideally, in a system where the MBBP coverage provided by both GHI and PHI is uniform and the price of premiums is readily apparent to all market segments, buyers of health insurance may choose between GHI and PHI based not only on philosophic preference, but also on price, service, reputation and convenience.

GHI presently pays fee-for-service for most of the medical services it buys but sets fees at a highly discounted rate. GHI could explore other payment options. Perhaps in the way that the Japanese healthcare cooperatives negotiate the costs, GHI could negotiate future costs and pass those costs, and all administrative costs, to all who have not enrolled in PHI (all who do not demonstrate evidence of having purchased PHI). Such an option would mean that the GHI health insurance premium would change each year reflecting estimated total costs for the coming year and would free GHI from dependence on relatively fixed tax revenues. Such a system of non-profit GHI healthcare cooperatives might prove to be stiff competition for PHI. The point being, there are plenty of options to be explored if a dynamic multi-payor system is preserved.

Once insurance became mandatory, enrollment in GHI would be the default choice; individuals would have to choose PHI intentionally. My belief is that the PHI industry would recognize the size of this market and compete aggressively for the whole of it. Shown below is Figure 7, which shows each segment of the market. Insured large business employees are shown on the left, hereafter referred to as the "PHI segment." Those enrolled in GHI are shown on the right, hereafter referred to as the "GHI segment." The shared market of small business employees, the privately insured, and the uninsured are shown in the center as a group, hereafter called the "shared segment."

Also shown in Figure 7 is the uninsured population divided into two segments. The segment that selects GHI is shown on the right of a diagonal line, while the segment that selects PHI is shown on the left of the diagonal line. This is not, of course, the only possible division of the shared segment between GHI and PHI.

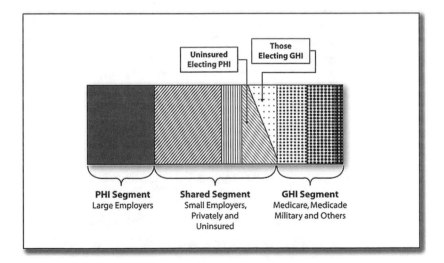

Figure 7: Alternative Distribution A

Alternative distributions between those who select GHI or PHI are shown in Figures 8 and 9. In Figure 8 a large proportion of the shared segment selects GHI. Such a distribution would imply that GHI had chosen a price competitive strategy to lower the price of health coverage for all and that GHI has enrolled large numbers of insurees from among small employers and those who are privately insured as well as the uninsured. In order to accomplish this, GHI must take advantage of its ability to keep management costs low and to set low fees for medical services.

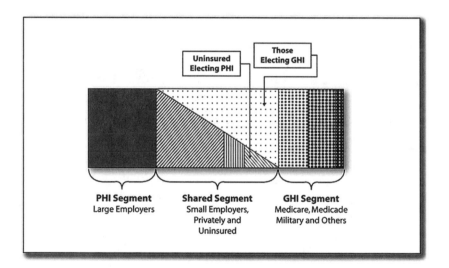

Figure 8: Alternative Distribution B

In the long run, low fees for medical services may fail to finance new infrastructure at a rate comparable to the rate at which a market driven system would invest in new infrastructure. Lower fees may discourage providers from accepting GHI patients. Lower fees and limited infrastructure ultimately result in soft rationing and under-utilization of services for all patients. Under-utilization of services may affect quality and outcomes.

In Figure 9 a smaller portion of the shared segment selects GHI. This is the version of the model most likely to survive. Considering the business, marketing and management skills of PHI, one can hardly imagine that PHI will be out-bid by GHI. Furthermore, PHI will provide choices, efficiencies, amenities and conveniences that GHI cannot provide.

In this model insurance premiums will be price sensitive; there will be market sensitivity for the medical services patients use; there will be funds flowing through the healthcare industry to build and renew facilities and other infrastructure. There may or may not be over-utilization of services.

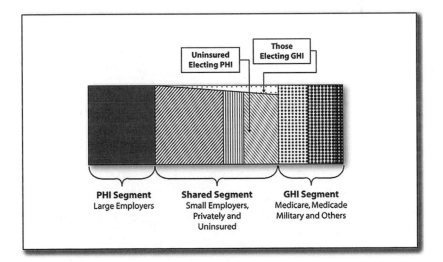

Figure 9: Alternative Distribution C

Conclusion

With this model, the entire population would have access to a uniform MBBP. The PHI segment (employees of large businesses) would have freedom to purchase insurance from any available insurance carrier. The shared segment would have its choice of any available insurance carrier or could choose GHI.

Any individual insurance provider would offer the MBBP at a single price to both the PHI segment and the shared segment, and no individual would be refused insurance. Those unwilling to purchase PHI would be enrolled by default in GHI and charged a premium. Insurance companies would compete based on price and service rather than their ability to identify risk

.

Other models are certainly feasible. This model determines eligibility for enrollment in GHI based on employer size. The Netherlands and Germany have made eligibility decisions based on income and the Japanese have made that decision based to some extent on occupation. The success of any multi-payor universal healthcare system apparently has less to do with the determination of which segments of the population are eligible for GHI than with correctly preserving a "normal" market for PHI.

CHAPTER THIRTEEN

And the Winners Are!

One day there will be universal healthcare in the United States.

One day a President of the United States will sign the bill that makes universal healthcare a reality.

Before that day, Congress will debate the bill. Congress will have determined that the proposal provides basic healthcare for all U.S. citizens and is sustainable. What will be in that bill?

What will make universal healthcare fiscally sustainable <u>and</u> politically palatable? Anyone could hammer together a list of healthcare benefits and hype them in a universal healthcare package. But making that package financially feasible — there's a real trick!

Today, more than forty-five million Americans have no healthcare coverage. The proportion of Americans who receive health insurance through their employment shrinks annually. Yet, there is no natural constituency for universal healthcare of any consequence. That is to say there are not enough uninsured voters to bother with; eighty-five percent of the population already has some form of healthcare coverage. Most of the uninsured are healthy and therefore have no immediate need to trouble themselves with health insurance. A small few of the uninsured are sick — too sick to make a fuss. Admittedly, a portion of the uninsured includes workers for low or part time wages; they are earners, but they do not earn enough to choose to purchase health insurance privately, nor do they earn enough to actively lobby for healthcare. The populations who need universal healthcare coverage are those who are least likely to ask for it.

Ironically, the largest constituency for universal healthcare should be persons who are already insured! It is this population, 85% of the people of this country, who — through the mechanism of cost-shifting — are already paying for the healthcare of the uninsured. This is the population that ought to advocate universal healthcare!

There are also substantial groups of educated and well-meaning people who understand the sad plight of the uninsured; they understand and feel the impact of going without needed medical services and of unnecessary premature deaths that result from lack of access to medical services. These are the devoted supporters of universal healthcare.

These groups provide the momentum for universal healthcare proposals; some do so for humanitarian or philosophical reasons and some for economic reasons. Together, they could have strong influence toward the passage of universal healthcare, but they are divided. They are divided in their beliefs about how the most favorable system for providing universal healthcare should be modeled, they are divided in their beliefs about how such a system should be paid for, and they are divided in their thoughts about how healthcare services should be distributed.

Some recommend a single-payor system, which generally implies a government managed system with authority to levy the necessary taxes to pay for healthcare services (and management and regulation); others prefer a heavily regulated multi-payor system with fixed prices or not-for-profit insurance companies. Some are willing to accept a tiered healthcare system; others insist that all healthcare services be available to all people regardless of ability to pay, insisting that healthcare is a "right." There is no shortage of strongly held opinion.

Before these groups become effective, there must be some agreement about what policy will be effective — about the dictates of pragmatism.

What will congress approve? What will a president sign? What will the uniquely American Universal Healthcare System look like?

Decision-making, especially political decision-making in the United States, is seldom purely objective. Political decisions are not always made according to the relative merits of the various alternatives. Rather, various positions are made in public debate, constituencies grow and shrink, and then decisions are made by votes. Objectivity will creep into and out of the debate, and as objectivity fluctuates, so will the prospect of a viable plan.

There are many factors to consider in designing a national healthcare system suitable to a population as large and as diverse as that of the United States. The goal has already proven elusive. It may already be too late for real objectivity — so many strongly held positions having already been staked on this particular field.

The purpose of this book has been to look at existing universal healthcare programs and examine their relative merits and failings, then to propose a foundation for a sustainable universal healthcare policy and system based on economic and business principles. The principles described here have been gleaned from the experiments and experiences of other countries.

One model has been proposed, but whatever model evolves, it should represent a workable, solvent, sustainable solution to universal healthcare in the U.S.

The multi-payor model proposed here may be nothing more than another page in the discussion about healthcare in the U.S., but those who have assisted in bringing this work to completion have done so with confidence that the discussion about basic economics remains important.

Those in the healthcare industry know that health insurance is not really "insurance," at least not when insurance is defined as protection against an unpredictable event. Rather, health insurance is a redistribution of the costs of two very predictable events, aging and disease. These events are inevitable. With a little luck,

> Health insurance is a redistribution of the costs of two very predictable events: aging and disease.

everyone will have the opportunity to "age," and few people die in perfect health. Health insurance under conditions of price differentiation is simply a process of graduated premiums; as these two inevitable events unfold, premiums go up and up, and in the end, many forego medical care because premium costs have become prohibitive.

But under conditions of community rating, a more even premium is paid throughout life; people have the opportunity to contribute earlier to cover the costs of healthcare before age and illness reduce the capacity to pay. And they retain coverage for catastrophic events that might occur during their younger years.

The first purpose of developing a universal healthcare policy is to assure healthcare benefits to all; it should not be neglected, however, that there are considerable social and economic benefits that follow universal healthcare.

For the United States to realize the secondary benefits associated with universal healthcare, government must initially mandate that everyone will be insured. If a multi-payor system is to succeed, government must then foster an environment conducive to competition based on price, convenience, amenities, and reputation rather than on administrative costs or risk. There must be a market with sufficiently large numbers of insurers to promote competition. And in order for insurers to truly compete based on price, insurers must be offered a level playing field; they must uniformly be required to offer the same minimum basic benefits policy, and they must be required to sell it to any who apply to purchase it.

Under the parameters of this particular model, a level playing field would allow insurance companies to continue as profitable enterprises. They will prosper as well in the United States as they do in other OECD member countries where community rating and guaranteed issue are mandatory. Without appropriate regulations, however, PHI cannot accomplish this policy role. Regulations must be in place simply to keep the playing field level.

If these conditions can be met, healthcare will be universally available and universally portable at a competitive market price. By assigning GHI the role of caring for vulnerable populations, and by protecting the role of PHI to insure employees of large companies, stable infrastructure for both GHI and PHI is assured. By asking GHI and PHI to share, and in a sense to compete for, the remaining market consisting of employees of small companies, the self-employed, and those currently uninsured, policy makers will assure universal access to healthcare coverage, either through default selection of GHI, or by active selection of either GHI or PHI.

By preserving market forces in the healthcare industry, the market driven impetus for innovation will continue to bring new technologies and new efficiencies to healthcare. The advantages of market distribution will be preserved in as much as possible. Consumer choice will be preserved. It is worth remembering that in countries where PHI is used as a policy tool, waiting lists for medical elective services are uncommon; access meets market demand, and solvency — which is related to the costs of doing business — is not dependent upon raising taxes!

America needs universal healthcare from an economic as well as from a moral point of view. Other nations have provided both universal healthcare and contained healthcare costs while doing so. Certainly Americans can find both the ingenuity and the political will to accomplish this necessary task.

Selvoy M. Fillerup, MD, MSPH, FACS

Appendix

I: Insurance v. Cost-shifting

It may be arguable that it is less efficient to redistribute healthcare costs after delivery of service than before delivery of services. After all, universal healthcare systems everywhere have lower total healthcare expenditures than we do in the U.S.: some countries spend 7 or 8% of GDP on healthcare; the U.S. spends 14.5%. True, some portion of that cost is attributable to managerial costs, or to over-utilization, but some portion of that cost must certainly be attributable to the infrastructure needed to administer the activities of cost-shifting.

Cost-shifting, performed after delivery of care, is performed as a secondary function within provider systems not built for, or intended for, that purpose. Cost-shifting is performed as a necessary afterthought. It is an expensive service. It is a cost center. How can hospitals ever charge for that service? It is an unnecessary economic burden, and its costs must also, of necessity, be passed on to insured patients.

I find it tempting to imagine myself as a board member of a health insurance company. Cost redistribution of medical care is my business. But cost-shifting is also the redistribution of costs of medical care. And hospitals are doing it! Hospitals are doing my business! Hospitals are redistributing the costs of medical services! I am outraged! And they are doing it badly. And they pass the cost of that activity to me and my clients!

Furthermore, they don't really want to be doing it. For hospitals and providers, cost-shifting is an expense; for insurance companies, cost redistribution is revenue. It is what insurers do. And with a couple of policy changes, insurers could have that business.

Insurers should want the government to make health insurance mandatory. Insurers should not want hospitals redistributing the costs of medical care for 15% of the population and then billing them, the insurers, for the effort! This should be insurance business.

II: Benefits Bundling v. Price Sensitivity

The OECD defines complementary and supplementary insurance differently than we do in the United States.

If a new U.S. healthcare policy defines MBBP and makes it mandatory for everyone to purchase this insurance, there will almost certainly be an immediate market for complementary and supplementary benefits packages. How the marketing of complementary and supplementary benefits affects the purchase of MBBP insurance will depend upon whether bundling of benefits packages is allowed.

It must be remembered that price sensitivity will be affected if bundling practices emerge that penalize insurees for switching carriers.

III: DALYs as a Surrogate Measure of Utilization

If over-utilization is to be contained by deductibles and co-payment, there will be a segment of the population who under-utilize preventive healthcare services, because for that segment, the amount of the co-payment will be prohibitively high. At least this will be the case if co-payments are uniform for all services and for all patients.

Over-utilization, under-utilization, and the concepts of quality and outcomes are linked in subtle ways to reimbursement for medical services. It is only natural that providers will, at least to some degree, tend to provide services for which they are well reimbursed.

In the U.S. we use a reimbursement system of calculated "Relative Value Scales" and "Diagnosis Related Groups" to determine the payments given for medical services. Absent from these calculations is any consideration of the level of community health gained by the service provided.

One standard measure of community health is the Disability Adjusted Life Year (DALY). DALYs were introduced in 1994 by Murray et al as a means of estimating the cost effectiveness and the improvement in community health in response to any given medical intervention. DALYs provide a means of comparison of both the health outcomes and the cost effectiveness of various interventions.[64]

If DALYs were included in the calculations of RVS and DRG scales, and if procedures proven to save DALYs were reimbursed at higher rates than services that had little or no effect on community health (for example an immunization paid at 90% of its fee vs. a tonsillectomy paid at 70% of its fee), providers could be expected to perform services for which a higher percentage of the fee was reimbursed.

In this manner, services that improved public health would be readily identified by their reimbursement rates, providers would have an incentive to perform evidence-based preventive healthcare measures, good population outcomes would thereby be reinforced, and that elusive measure Quality of Care might come within reach. DALYs are, after all, measurable.[65]

IV. Regarding Risk Ratings, Price Discrimination, and Universal Healthcare

A fox chasing two rabbits catches neither.

--Folk saying

In a recent conversation about universal healthcare, a friend spoke of his concerns about the cost of financing healthcare and said he had come to the conclusion that individuals who engage in behaviors that increased the likelihood that they would have increased healthcare costs ought to pay more for healthcare coverage. In other words, people who engage in risky behaviors should be made to pay more. I told him I understood his position, but I disagreed.

The goal of enacting universal healthcare in the United States has been elusive for decades. It is true that financing universal healthcare has been a major hurdle. But, coupling the financing of universal healthcare with other agendas can only compromise the achievement of the primary goal — providing universal healthcare.

The characteristics of a multi-payor universal healthcare plan based on a uniform minimum basic benefits package (MBBP) and community ratings have been previously described. Such a plan would bring some degree of market efficiency to the health insurance market and would eliminate the prohibitive insurance premiums associated with price discrimination for many citizens with pre-existing medical conditions.

Others, besides this friend, have suggested that risk ratings with higher priced premiums for individuals with high-risk occupations, or high-risk behaviors, are appropriate and necessary in order to successfully finance universal healthcare. Although health risks associated with behavior or occupation or genetics do affect healthcare costs, these risk patterns are, in reality, issues separate from the issue of universal healthcare.

High-risk occupations, high-risk behaviors and genetic risks deserve to be addressed separately for the following reasons:

- *Any group considered at higher risk for any reason-- genetic risk, occupational risk, or pre-existing medical condition--will have cause to express political opposition to any universal healthcare plan financed in part by risk ratings.*

- *Community ratings in the insurance industry would compel or persuade policy makers to consider other risk factors as independent problems, rather than in terms of how those problems affect health insurance.*

- *Risky behaviors such as smoking are inherently different from health risks related to genetic causes.*

- *It is sophomoric to assume that variation in the price of insurance premiums will provide remedies for either type of risk. (Policy makers ought to consider tobacco use in one forum and genetic diseases in another forum.)*

- *The definitions of "risk" will surely change over time.*

- *Policy makers would have to change risk-rating criteria with each new development that placed any one group at higher risk than any other group, and would have to address political opposition each time there was a change in the definition of risk.*

- *The consequence would be that at-risk individuals with the greatest political influence would pay the least for insurance, while those with limited political influence would pay the most.[66]*

- *Once risk ratings are allowed for one reason, they may be allowed for any number of reasons.*

  - *This would eliminate the market benefits associated with community ratings.*

  - *Risk rating practices have already placed health insurance out of reach for individuals with pre-existing medical conditions and would continue to do so.*

Establishing a universal healthcare system in the United States should be considered as a single issue. Other issues that affect healthcare costs are, in reality, separate issues, and should be considered on the basis of finding specific solutions to those problems, rather than expecting them to be magically solved by increasing healthcare premiums.

Focused methods of addressing individual at-risk populations will produce solutions expressly tailored to those populations. (For example, if the long-term goal is to improve health and lower healthcare costs by reducing tobacco consumption, taxing tobacco is more likely to have an effect than increasing rates for health insurance. Nor do I believe that price discrimination for health insurance will alter any risk-taking behavior in any significant way!)

Rather, linking increased health risks for any reason whatever to increased premiums invites other forms of price discrimination, and ultimately invites political opposition to universal healthcare--especially from those who would pay the highest premiums.

Any universal healthcare policy should focus primarily on healthcare, and should not become a vehicle for social tasks for which it is not designed.

Remember: *A fox chasing two rabbits catches neither.*

V. Oversight

In their book <u>Critical Condition,</u> authors Bartlett and Steele suggest that oversight of healthcare policy be given to an organization patterned after the Federal Reserve Bank — the Fed.[67] They even suggest a title, "United States Commission on Health Care," the US-CHC. Their recommendation is a good one. Their reasons include the fact that the Fed is able to act on its own agenda without fear of direct political pressure from either the Executive or the Legislative branches of government. This is so because the board members are appointed for fourteen-year terms. The added benefit of these long-term appointments is that the institution has "memory" — members on its board with years of insight into past problems and solutions.

The Fed's website is instructive. The site reveals a long list of departments and duties that fall under the Fed's umbrella. In a flash it becomes apparent that just such an organization is needed to accomplish the enormous agenda of implementing universal multi-payor healthcare in the United States.

The Fed is responsible for investigating and enforcing several aspects of monetary policy. The following information, for example, comes from the Fed's web site:

"The Federal Reserve supervises the following entities and has the statutory authority to take formal enforcement actions against them:

- *State member banks*
- *Bank holding companies*

- *Non-bank subsidiaries of bank holding companies*

- *Edge and agreement corporations*

- *Branches and agencies of foreign banking organizations operating in the United States and their parent banks*

- *Officers, directors, employees, and certain other categories of individuals associated with the above banks, companies, and organizations (referred to as "institution-affiliated parties")*

Generally, the Federal Reserve takes formal enforcement actions against the above entities for violations of laws, rules, or regulations, unsafe or unsound practices, breaches of fiduciary duty, and violations of final orders. Formal enforcement actions include cease and desist orders, written agreements, removal and prohibition orders, and orders assessing civil money penalties. (http://www.federalreserve.gov/boarddocs/enforcement/)

It only makes sense that a US-CHC would have similar responsibilities regarding healthcare and the oversight of performance and compliance of insurance providers. Just as the United States' financial markets benefit from having banks of differing sizes and structures, the country's health insurance market likewise benefits from having insurance providers with differing size and structure. And just as the Fed sets interest rates, the US-CHC will have a responsibility to set premium rates for GHI. Those rates will profoundly affect the prices of PHI premiums.

It would be imperative that the US-CHC have oversight of all of GHI and that the business of GHI be transparent and function as nearly as possible as if it were a competing insurance company. After all, if GHI is allowed to rely too heavily on taxation for revenues, it could destroy PHI. (That particular scenario is unlikely; Americans will hardly encourage tax increases for any purpose, but the need for oversight remains.)

Regional variation in insurance markets is another area of concern. The price of health insurance is surely different in California than in Mississippi. There may be regional variations in GHI premium prices that will have effects on PHI markets. Likewise, the percentage of the population electing enrollment in GHI rather than PHI will vary by region.

The solvency of PHI providers must be assured. This is largely a state function under current systems, but a national healthcare policy could change the nature of that function. Just as the Fed performs both regulatory and protective functions for banks, a US-CHC would provide regulatory and protective functions for the insurance industry.

The US-CHC must also enforce the regulations for community ratings, guaranteed issue, and a uniform MBBP, and assure that bundling of benefits packages does not impair market competition.

In short, there is plenty for a US-CHC to do without becoming — indeed to avoid becoming — a monolithic single-payor entity. One purpose of establishing a multi-payor universal healthcare system is to avoid the problems faced by single-payor systems and capture the benefits of market economies in healthcare. We are, after all, speaking of an industry that presently accounts for 14% of U.S. GDP. If it is our intent to improve upon that number, and to protect both public and private interests in the process, it is imperative to have an organization with the agenda to do so. Without a US-CHC, universal healthcare in a multi-payor environment cannot succeed.

Selvoy M. Fillerup, MD, MSPH, FACS

Reference List

1. Evans, RG. (2005). Fellow Travelers on a Contested Path: Power, Purpose, and the Evolution of European Health Care Systems. *Journal of Health Politics, Policy and Law. 30*, 277-294.

2. Institutes of Medicine of the National Academies. The Uninsured Are Sicker and Die Sooner. Available at: http://www.iom.edu/Object.File/Master/17/748/ Fact%20sheet%205%20Quality.pdf.

3. Associated Press. <u>About 2 million more Americans uninsured</u> (June 25, 2007) [Web Page]. URL http:// www.azcentral.com/news/articles/ 0625uninsured0625-ON.html [accessed 2007, July 10].

4. Colombo F, and Tapay, N. (2004). Private Health Insurance in OECD Countries: The Benefits and Costs for Individuals and Health Systems. OECD Health Working Papers No. 15. Available at: http:// www.oecd.org/dataoecd/34/56/33698043.pdf

5. Cotis, JP. (2003). Healthcare demand in Europe: Economic growth and sustainability of the European Model. The Europe of Health, EFPIA Annual Meeting

2003, Athens. Paris: Organisation for Economic Cooperation and Development. Available at: http://www.oecd.org/dataoecd/34/56/33698043.pdf

6. US Census Bureau, US Department of Commerce, Economics and Statistics Administration. Life Expectancy and Rates of Infant Mortality. Available at: http://www.census.gov/cgi-bin/ipc/idbsprd.

7. Kaiser Commission on Medicaid and the Uninsured. (2004). Health Insurance Coverage in America. Washington, D.C.: The Henry J. Kaiser Family Foundation. Available at: http://www.kff.org/uninsured/upload/Health-Coverage-in-America-2004-Data-Update-Report.pdf

8. HMO profits increase 10.7% in 2004. (2005, August). South Florida Business Journal, August 8, 2005; accessed December 27, 2005. Web Page. Available at: http://www.bizjournals.com/industries/health_care/health_insurance/2005/08/08/orlando_daily2.html?.

9. Institutes of Medicine of the National Academies. The Uninsured Are Sicker and Die Sooner. Available at: http://www.iom.edu/Object.File/Master/17/748/Fact%20sheet%205%20Quality.pdf.

10. Schoen C, Osborn R, Huynh PT, et al.(2005). Taking the Pulse of Health Care Systems: Experiences of Patients with Health Problems in Six Countries. *Health Affairs Web Exclusive*, 509-525.

11. Colombo F, and Tapay, N. (2004). Private Health Insurance in OECD Countries: The Benefits and

Costs for Individuals and Health Systems. OECD Health Working Papers No. 15. Available at: http://www.oecd.org/dataoecd/34/56/33698043.pdf

12. Organisation for Economic Cooperation and Development: OECD Health Project. (2004). Proposal for a Taxonomy of Health Insurance. *OECD Study on Private Health Insurance.*

13. Sbarbaro, JA. (2000). Trade Liberalization in Health Insurance: Opportunities and Challenges: The Potential Impact of Introducing or Expanding the Availability of Private Health Insurance Within Low and Middle Income Countries. WHO Commission on Macroeconomics and Health. Available at: http://www.cmhealth.org/docs/wg4_paper6.pdf

14. OECD. (2004). Health Systems Must Seek Better Value for Money, OECD Concludes in Report to Health Ministers. Available at: http://www.oecd.org/document/26/0,2340,en_2649_33929_31734042_1_1_1_1,00.html.

15. Tuohy C.H., Flood C.M., Stabile M. (2004). How Does Private Finance Affect Public Health Care Systems? Marshaling the Evidence from OECD Nations. *Journal of Health Politics, Policy and Law. 29*, 359-396.

16. Top court strikes down Quebec private health-care ban. (2005, June 9). *www.cbc.ca.* Available at: http://www.cbc.ca/story/canada/national/2005/06/09/newscoc-health050609.html.

17. Unsocialized Medicine, A landmark ruling exposes Canada's health-care inequity. (2005, June 13). *The*

Wall Street Journal. Available at: http:// www.opinionjournal.com/editorial/ feature.html?id=110006813.

18. Knappe, Eckhard. (2005). A Healthcare Market for Europe? accessed April 4, 2005. *Pfizer.* Available at: http://www.pfizerforum.com/english/knappe.shtml.

19. Docteur E, Oxley H. (2003). Health-Care Systems: Lessons From the Reform Experience. *OECD Health Working Papers. 9.* Available at: http:// www.oecd.org/dataoecd/5/53/22364122.pdf

20. DeCoster C. (2002). Measuring and managing waiting times: what's to be done? *Health Manage Forum. 15,* 6-10, 46-50.

21. McGurran J, Noseworthy T. (2002). Improving the management of waiting lists for elective healthcare services: public perspectives on proposed solutions. *Hosp Q. 5,* 28-32.

22. Shortt SE, Shaw RA, Elliott D, Mackillop WJ. (2004). Monitoring trends in waiting periods in Canada for elective surgery: validation of a method using administrative data. *Can J Surg. 47,* 173-8.

23. Protti DJ. Canada's Federated Healthcare System; A Past, Present and Future View. *Health Care Systems in Flux: The Case of Canada and the United States.* Seminar conducted at The University of Colorado at Denver and Health Sciences Center, Denver, Colorado.

24. Greengross P , Grant K, Collini E. (1999). *The History and Development of The UK National Health Service*

1948 - 1999. (2nd ed.) London: Department of International Development Health Systems Resource Centre.

25. Damiani M, Propper C, Dixon J. (2005).Mapping choice in the NHS: cross sectional study of routinely collected data. *BMJ. 330,* 284.

26. Duckett SJ. (2005).Private care and public waiting. *Aust Health Rev. 29,* 87-93.

27. Dusheiko M, Gravelle H, Jacobs R. (2004). The effect of practice budgets on patient waiting times: allowing for selection bias. *Health Econ. 13,* 941-58.

28. Dodds W, Morgan M, Wolfe C, Raju KS. (2004). Implementing the 2-week wait rule for cancer referral in the UK: general practitioners' views and practices. *Eur J Cancer Care (Engl). 13,* 82-7.

29. Gravelle H, Sutton M, Morris S, et al. (2003). Modelling supply and demand influences on the use of health care: implications for deriving a needs-based capitation formula. *Health Econ. 12,* 985-1004.

30. Siciliani L, Hurst J. (2005). Tackling excessive waiting times for elective surgery: a comparative analysis of policies in 12 OECD countries. *Health Policy. 72,* 201-15.

31. Grant, Sue. (n.d.). Healthcare in Germany. Available at: http://www.medhunters.com/articles/healthcareInGermany.html.

32. Gordeeva, Tatyana. (1998).German Culture; Health Insurance. Available at: http://

www.germanculture.com.ua/library/facts/
bl_health_insurance.htm.

33. Ikegami N, Campbell JC. (2004). Japan's health care system: containing costs and attempting reform. *Health Aff (Millwood). 23*, 26-36.

34. Kawabuchi, Koichi. (2004, April). Features of Japan's Healthcare system. Available at: http:// www.jijigaho.or.jp/app/0404/eng/sp08.html.

35. Koopmanschap MA, Brouwer WB, Hakkaart-van Roijen L, van Exel NJ. (2005). Influence of waiting time on cost-effectiveness. *Soc Sci Med. 60*, 2501-4.

36. Oudhoff JP, Timmermans DR, Bijnen AB, van der Wal G. (2004). Waiting for elective general surgery: physical, psychological and social consequences. *ANZ J Surg. 74*, 361-7.

37. Rexius H, Brandrup-Wognsen G, Oden A, Jeppsson A. (2004). Mortality on the waiting list for coronary artery bypass grafting: incidence and risk factors. *Ann Thorac Surg. 77*, 769-74; discussion 774-5.

38. MacCormick AD, Parry BR. (2003). Waiting time thresholds: are they appropriate? *ANZ J Surg. 73*, 926-8.

39. Ensor T, Cooper S. (2004). Overcoming barriers to health service access: influencing the demand side. *Health Policy Plan. 19*, 69-79.

40. Simantov E, Schoen C, Breugman S. (2001). Market Failure? Individual Insurance Markets for Older Americans. *Health Affairs. 20*, 139-149.

41. Sbarbaro, JA. (2000). Trade Liberalization in Health Insurance: Opportunities and Challenges: The Potential Impact of Introducing or Expanding the Availability of Private Health Insurance Within Low and Middle Income Countries. WHO Commission on Macroeconomics and Health. Available at: http://www.cmhealth.org/docs/wg4_paper6.pdf

42. Woolhandler S, Campbell T, Himmelstein D. (2003). Costs of Health Care Administration in the United States and Canada. *The New England Journal of Medicine. 349,* 768-775.

43. Cotis, JP. (2003). Healthcare Demand in Europe: Economic Growth and Sustainability of the European Model. Paris, France: Organisation for Economic Cooperation and Development.

44. Schenk, R. (2002). Insurance. Available at: http://ingrimayne.saintjoe.edu/econ/RiskExclusion/Risk.html.

45. Bhandari, S. (2004). People With Health Insurance: A Comparison of Estimates From Two Surveys. Washington, D.C.: U.S. Department of Commerce, U.S. Census Bureau.

46. US Census Bureau, US Department of Commerce, Economics and Statistics Administration. (n.d.) Health Insurance Coverage, Census Bureau Survey of Income and Program Participation, U.S. Census Bureau. Health Insurance Coverage: Who had a Lapse Between 1991 and 1993. Available at: http://www.census.gov/apsd/www/statbrief/sb95_21.pdf.

47. Fillerup, SM. (2005, Nov. 22). Should the United States Adopt a Single-payor or a Multi-payor Universal Healthcare Model? Available at: http://www.signalhealth.com/node/492/.

48. Cox, S. (2004, Oct. 21). What the Left Doesn't Get: The Small Business Lobby's Big Issues. *Counterpunch.* Available at: http://www.counterpunch.org/cox10212004.html.

49. U.S. Department of Labor, Office of Disability Employment Policy. (n.d.) Small Business and Self Employment for People with Disabilities. Available at: http://www.dol.gov/odep/pubs/ek00/small.htm.

50. Levitt, JC. (2004, Summer). Transfer of financial risk and alternative financing solutions. *J Health Care Finance. 30,* 21-32.

51. Durenburger, D. (2005). The 21st Century Health System: Integrated Systems and the Promise of Physician Leadership. Available at: www.nihp.org/Reports/21stCenturySummary.doc.

52. Lavigne, JE, Phelps, CE, Mushlin, A, Lednar, WM. (2003). Reductions in individual work productivity associated with type 2 diabetes mellitus. *Pharmacoeconomics. 21,* 1123-34.

53. Stewart, WF, Ricci, JA, Chee, E, Hahn, SR, Morganstein, D. (2003). Cost of lost productive work time among US workers with depression. *JAMA. 289,* 3135-44.

54. Wang, PS, Beck, AL, Berglund, P, et al. (2004). Effects of major depression on moment-in-time work performance. *Am J Psychiatry. 161,* 1885-91.

55. Vijan, S, Hayward, RA, Langa, KM. (2004). The impact of diabetes on workforce participation: results from a national household sample. *Health Serv Res. 39,* 1653-69.

56. Lerner, D, Adler, DA, Chang, H, et al. (2004). The clinical and occupational correlates of work productivity loss among employed patients with depression. *J Occup Environ Med. 46,* S46-55.

57. Stewart, WF, Ricci, JA, Chee, E, Morganstein, D, Lipton, R. (2003). Lost productive time and cost due to common pain conditions in the US workforce. *JAMA. 290,* 2443-54.

58. Lerner, D, Amick, BC, Lee, JC, et al. (2003). Relationship of employee-reported work limitations to work productivity. *Med Care. 41,* 649-59.

59. Ng, YC, Jacobs, P, Johnson, JA. (2001). Productivity losses associated with diabetes in the US. *Diabetes Care.* 24, 257-61.

60. Ramsey, S, Summers, KH, Leong, SA, Birnbaum, HG, Kemner, JE, Greenberg, P. (2002). Productivity and medical costs of diabetes in a large employer population. *Diabetes Care. 25,* 23-9.

61. Bramley, TJ, Lerner, D, Sames, M. (2002). Productivity losses related to the common cold. *J Occup Environ Med. 44,* 822-9.

62. Gallup, J, Sachs, JD. (2001). The Economic burden of malaria. *Am. J. Trop. Med. Hyg.* *64*(1,2 S), 85-96.

63. Buchmueller, TC , Grumbach K , Kronick R , Kahn JG. (2005). The effect of health insurance on medical care utilization and implications for insurance expansion: a review of the literature. *Med Care Res Rev.* *62*(1), 3-30.

64. Murray, C, Lopez, A, Jamison, D. (1994). The Global burden of disease in 1990: summary results, sensitivity analysis and future directions. *Bulletin of the World Health Organization.* *72*(3), 495-509.

65. McKenna, MT, Michaud, CM, Murray, CJL, Marks, JS. (2005). Assessing the Burden of Disease in the United States Using Disability-Adjusted Life Years. *Am J Prev Med.* *28*(5), 415-423.

66. Evans, RG. (1997). Going for the gold: the redistributive agenda behind market-based health care reform. *J Health Polit Policy Law.* *22*, 427-65.

67. Bartlett, DL, Steele, JB. *Critical Condition.* New York: Doubleday; 2004.

For further information about Multi-payor Universal Healthcare Systems, to purchase additional copies of this book, or to contact the author, please visit the website www.selvoyfillerup.com

Index

A

B

C

D

E

F

G

H

R

S

T

U

To contact Dr Fillerup, to schedule him as a speaker to your civic, social, or political group, or to purchase additional copies of *Chronic Crisis*, visit chroniccrisis.com or contact the publisher.